30 DAY

MENTAL HEALTH BOOT CAMP

Kristin Stonesifer, LCSW

30 DAY

MENTAL HEALTH BOOT CAMP

30 days to a better, stronger, healthier you

Learn the skills professionals use to become your own therapist

Contents

Acknowledgements

This book would not be as extraordinary as it is without the incredible contribution of Carol A. Kirby. To have someone as passionate about your vision for a book is a rare gift that most authors only dream about. Wherever this book is articulate and elegant, it is most likely due to her attention to detail and mastery with articulating a point or concept. To her I owe a debt of gratitude I may never be able to repay.

I would also like to acknowledge the thousands of incredible people I have worked with in my career who inspired and influenced the making of this book. I am continually inspired by the courage of strangers to open up the deepest parts of their soul to a complete stranger and allow me into their private worlds. It takes incredible strength to ask for mental health help, given the stigma that still exists. I cannot impress upon my clients enough the impact that they have had on me to discover my own courage. Without my many clients and patients over the years, this book would not be possible, and to them I owe a debt of gratitude I may never be able to repay.

Lastly and most importantly, I would like to thank my father who departed this world in 2013. He taught me the most important belief that is woven into my very being: anything is possible. John Wirth was a dreamer. He never let failure stop him or even slow him down. He viewed failure as a learning process and I was lucky enough to witness his fortitude first hand. He taught me a love of the English language and the power of being able to communicate a sentiment and a feeling with just the right word. His unconditional love solidified what would have otherwise been a shaky foundation and I am grateful that God chose him to be my father. I miss him dearly every day and I dedicate this book to his memory and in his honor. I love you, Dad. I hope you are proud of your TT.

Introduction

Good mental health does not have to be as complicated as we make it. So many tools that are effective are not taught to us, and are often not modeled by our primary caretakers. My goal for this book is to put forth the most effective, important tools to start you on a path of good mental health.

I am perpetually frustrated by the continuing stigma of mental health and the fear of admitting our emotional struggles. Individuals experience a tremendous pressure to conceal their difficulties and their mental health illnesses. We never hesitate to mention an aching back or sore throat, but rarely admit, "my anxiety is high today!"

Our mental health is something we experience every day, much like managing our physical well-being. Schools teach physical health, our parents teach us information about our bodies, magazines and the internet are full of articles about physical well-being, but mental health is still in the dark ages. We never learn how to manage and treat our mental health, whether it is recognizing and addressing an issue, or learning what we can do to strengthen and improve good mental health. Most people unnecessarily suffer in silence for many years and only seek mental health help when they reach a breaking point. Many people don't know what they are struggling with, especially with posttraumatic stress disorder.

Of the information that is available, most of it assists with identifying the problem. Very little information actually provides the tools needed to remediate the issue. Most articles have some form of "Do you struggle with any of these symptoms?" for the title, which helps people with problem identification. But just like diagnosing a problem with your car, it doesn't do much good until you fix the problem. As far as coping skills, they are akin to putting duct tape on a rattle in your car. It may stop the noise for a while, but it won't fix the problem.

My goal with writing this book is to give people useful skills to begin to resolve their mental health issues. Beyond understanding the actual issue at hand, the why and the how are the keys to healing.

The idea for this book came as I pondered the best way to share the most effective tools I use with my clients in a more prolific manner. As much as I enjoy working with my clients and helping one person at a time, my goal as a mental health professional is to help as many people as possible with eliminating mental suffering in order to lead extraordinary lives. My goal was to develop a format that is practical and easy to use, but effective and inspirational.

Fixing broken mental health can be overwhelming. This book is broken down into one day at a time, which is the best way to manage an overwhelming task when you don't know where to begin. Each day covers a separate topic and is designed in a specific order. Homework assignments are crucial to incorporating the concepts covered for the day. Just like any other task we undertake, you will get out of this book what you put into it.

I hope these skills help you to live a happy, full life, as much as they have helped me.

Author's Note

    This book is designed to cover credible and helpful information regarding basic mental health concepts. It is offered with the intention that the author is not rendering clinical assistance in place of therapeutic intervention. If additional assistance or therapy is needed, contact a licensed professional in your area.

DAY 1 ABC WORKSHEETS

Today is an exciting day as you begin this journey. Not only is it the first day, but it is an important day. All of the Boot Camp lessons are useful but today's lesson is, without a doubt, the most powerful and important, hence making it the topic of Day 1. It is a long lesson, so stick with it. You won't regret it! Once you understand ABC worksheets and the cognitive process, you will possess the most helpful skill in your mental health tool belt.

Let's get started!

Today's Objective: 1) Be able to identify emotions 2) Learn the cognitive process in order to better manage emotions without "coping skills" 3) Begin to reframe the way you think

People usually do one of two things with emotions: they avoid them or they "circle the drain" with them. To escape painful or unpleasant emotions, people use evading behaviors that consist of either numbing behaviors or avoiding behaviors. Examples of these behaviors include alcohol or drug use, shopping, watching television, playing on cell phones, being promiscuous or distracting themselves with a romantic relationship, completely avoiding anxiety-producing situations, or an assortment of addictive behaviors.

Circling the drain involves allowing the emotion to overwhelm you, resulting in behaviors such as staying in bed all day, not showering, not getting help for mental health issues, remaining in abusive relationships (not an easy task to leave abusive situations), or just becoming one with the negative emotion.

Fortunately, there is a third option that does not involve merely coping, which, in essence, is an avoidance tactic. Managing or resolving the emotion is a much healthier solution. This lesson will teach you the cognitive process which leads to management or resolution using a method called ABC worksheets.

ABC worksheets are a powerful tool used in Cognitive Behavioral Therapy ("CBT"). Most psychotherapy performed today uses CBT techniques. When you go to a therapist for a session and talk, this technique is most likely what they are using while you are talking; they are identifying where your thought processes are distorted or negative. It is incredibly transformative when you begin utilizing it in your own life.

How many times have you said or heard someone say, "I can't help how I feel" or "she made me angry/mad/sad." We actually *can* help how we feel; we have more control over our emotions than we think we do. The following worksheets are the most important skill you will learn in this Boot Camp. Practice the worksheets *daily* until you learn the process. Once you have the process down, you will carry a very powerful tool in your mind at all times! The key to any tool is to remember to use it. When you practice using it, the process will become a natural one.

To begin, we will review two examples, then you can use the blank worksheet for your own situations. Make copies of the blank worksheet before you fill it in so that you have extras.

Instructions

Read the instructions first in order to understand the various sections, then read "Putting It All Together" to fully understand the process.

How the Worksheet Is Set Up

<u>Situation</u>

Notice that "Situation" goes straight across the top. Situations are events that occur. Events that happen to us cannot be changed. I cannot change that someone was abused as a child and I cannot change the event of a car accident. A situation can also be a behavior, such as someone saying something to us or something that someone does.

Situation:		
	Unhelpful	Helpful
Thoughts: *(I am…….)*		
Emotions/ Feelings		
Physical:		
Action/Behavior:		

<u>Thoughts</u>

The next section below Situation is "Thoughts." Thoughts are how we interpret the situation, what we think about the situation in terms of what we say to ourselves about ourselves. Thoughts are often automatic and we may not be conscious of them.

However, there is a trick to discovering our thoughts that you will learn!

Situation:		
	Unhelpful	Helpful
Thoughts: *(I am.......)*		
Emotions/ Feelings		
Physical:		
Action/Behavior:		

Emotions

After Thoughts is "Emotions or Feelings." Our thoughts drive the way we feel. When we adjust our thoughts, our feelings change. This mechanism is how we control our emotions. If I tell myself that I'm ugly, no one will ever love me, I'm going to die alone, how will I feel? Pretty depressed, right?

If I tell myself that I am beautiful, I am worthy of love, I have a very important purpose in my life right now, the right person will come along when the time is right, I will feel much differently, won't I? Now I feel grateful and empowered!

The goal of managing emotions is not necessarily to create a positive emotion. There are situations where you obviously will not feel happy. The goal is to either eliminate or weaken negative emotions. It is important to learn to tolerate feeling negative emotions. It is also important to remember that emotions are temporary. The purpose of learning this skill is to lessen the intensity and duration of negative emotions and train the brain to think more neutrally or positively. We are more productive and we engage the world more frequently and more effectively when we feel positive.

Situation:		
	Unhelpful	Helpful
Thoughts: *(I am.......)*		
Emotions/ Feelings		
Physical:		
Action/Behavior:		

Physical

After Emotions is "Physical." Physical responses occur simultaneously with the situation and the emotion. The purpose of this section is to identify what is physiologically going on in the body. What does my body physically feel like? This step is very helpful for anxiety and anger because those emotions are often accompanied by physical manifestations. Once you become more in touch with your physiological responses, your mind and body connection will strengthen and you can engage the cognitive process before your physiological responses become too intense.

Situation:		
	Unhelpful	Helpful
Thoughts: *(I am……..)*		
Emotions/ Feelings		
Physical:		
Action/Behavior:		

Action/Behavior

The "Action/Behavior" step refers to the resulting action. What did I do in response to the situation? As you learn the sequence of situation-thought-emotion and begin to master your emotional responses, your physiological responses will reduce in intensity and possibly subside, as will your reactive behaviors. You will become less *reactive* and more *responsive* as you master this skill and feel more in control of yourself.

Situation:		
	Unhelpful	Helpful
Thoughts: *(I am........)*		
Emotions/ Feelings		
Physical:		
Action/Behavior:		

<u>Unhelpful/Helpful Column</u>

The goal of the worksheet is to identify negative and distorted thoughts, challenge them, and replace them with more accurate and helpful thoughts. You will start in the unhelpful column, complete the unhelpful column, and then shift to the helpful column. For example, if my partner ends a romantic relationship with me (situation), an unhelpful way of thinking about the situation would be to tell myself that I'm unlovable, I'm going to be alone forever, and no one will ever want me again. How am I going to feel? Depressed and sad! If I tell myself that the relationship ran its course, I will learn something important from this experience, he/she is missing out because I'm awesome, and I will find the right person for me some day, then I will have a much more positive emotional response.

Situation:		
	Unhelpful	**Helpful**
Thoughts: *(I am…… ..)*		
Emotions/ Feelings		
Physical:		
Action/Behavior:		

Putting It All Together

When completing the worksheet, first identify the situation you wish to analyze. *NOTE: when you choose a situation, do not choose the death of a loved one that is related to the normal grieving process. It is normal to be sad over the loss of my elderly grandmother.*

Choose a situation and identify the behavior involved. A behavior is something that happens. Be specific. If it involves another person, identify what the person did or didn't do, said or didn't say. For example, "My husband didn't respond to my text message." "My husband is selfish" is not a situation, it is a criticism. Thus, identify the act, the behavior, or the statement which generated a strong reaction from you.

Next, skip *Thoughts* for now. Go to *Emotions*. Use the word list on page 17 to identify every single emotion associated with the *Situation*. Don't just pick the most intense 3 or 4 words. There is tremendous power and healing in putting precise words to what you feel. Often, a single situation can generate thirty emotions.

In situations, we can generally identify the emotions we feel, but we may not know what we are thinking or how we are interpreting the situation.

After you identify all of your emotions regarding the situation, go back to the *Thoughts* section.

1. Situation:		
	Unhelpful	Helpful
3. Thoughts: *(I am.........)*		
2. Emotions/ Feelings		
Physical:		
Action/Behavior:		

A Word About Thoughts

Our goal for Thoughts is to identify what we say *to ourselves about ourselves*. You are going to use a technique called "drilling down." Your initial interpretation about a situation may be about someone else, such as "He doesn't care about me." Drill down on the thought. In other words, ask yourself why you interpret the situation that way and specifically what does your interpretation say about you?

Get down to the "I am...." statement and away from the he/she statement directed at others.

For example, "He doesn't care about me" drills down to "I am not worth caring about."

The Trick to Identifying Thoughts

Here's the trick: look at the emotions you listed. Those words are clues to what you are thinking. Use the emotions listed to discover what you are saying to yourself. For example, if I write down an emotion of 'worthless,' that means I am telling myself (my thought) that I have no value or worth. If I feel inadequate, I am telling myself (my thought) I am worthy of being thrown away or I am not good enough.

Again, it is important to be specific and thorough when listing your emotions because the emotions hold a lot of information about ourselves.

The emotions we feel hold the key to our thoughts.

Completing the Worksheet

So, the *actual* order of our cognitive process is:

Situation – Thoughts – Feelings

but we complete the worksheet in the order of:

Situation – Feelings – Thoughts

Physical

The Physical section is used to identify what my body feels like. Some examples of physiological responses include stomach pains, physical tension, headache, clenched jaw, hands balled into fists, or low energy.

Action/Behavior

The Action/Behavior section is used to identify my resulting behavior. What am I doing in response to the situation? Examples include arguing, shutting down, walking away, drug or alcohol use, or using sarcasm.

A Word about Helpful Thoughts

After you have identified your unhelpful thoughts, the next step is to challenge them and create a new, more helpful interpretation of the situation. Day 6 will provide a more detailed way of challenging thoughts and beliefs that will further your mastery of this skill.

As you begin changing unhelpful thoughts, it is common to struggle with identifying a helpful thought. Look at the unhelpful thought. Your thought is most likely something negative about yourself that you believe is true. Often, we regard our thoughts and beliefs as true because there is a strong emotion associated with it. Habitually, we accept our automatic thoughts as accurate without challenging them. In fact, we may have difficulty accepting, as true, the helpful version of a negative thought.

Write it down anyway.

New thoughts and beliefs may feel weird at first. This feeling is normal. As you make your way through this Boot Camp, those new thoughts will begin to feel less awkward and, hopefully, will eventually begin to feel normal!

Let's look at some examples to demonstrate the cognitive process:

REJECTION EXAMPLE

Situation:	I'm at the big box store, walking down the aisle and someone I know walks by and does not acknowledge me.	
	Unhelpful	**Helpful**
Thoughts: *(I am……..)*	He/she ignored me. They don't like me. I am not likeable.	He/she looks a bit wrapped up in themselves. I wonder if there is something wrong? It's not personal. I'm ok. My value and worth does not depend on how others treat me or what others think of me.
Emotions/ Feelings	Low, sad, rejected	Concern
Physical:	Stomach cramps, low energy, feel sick	None, feel comfortable
Action/Behavior:	Go home and avoid them.	Get in touch and make sure they are ok.

In the first example, the event that has occurred (Situation) is *I am shopping at the big box store and someone I know walks by and does not acknowledge me.*

My immediate thought is that *they ignored me.*

That may be true! However, we need to "drill down" to the "I am" statement.

Why would someone ignore me?

They might ignore me if *they don't like me.*

That may be true! Why wouldn't someone like me?

Because *I am not a likeable person.* I am not a likeable person is one of my deep-down, core beliefs that came from somewhere else in my life, but I own it like it belongs to me!

Because of that belief, I feel *low, sad, rejected.*

The rejection comes from thinking that I am not a likeable person, not from the situation. We simply used the situation to confirm what we already believed to be true.

I have a physiological response of *stomach cramps, low energy, feeling sick.*

My behavioral response is to *go home and avoid the person.*

Now we need to reframe the thought. There is no room in my life for believing (the belief) that I am not a likeable person.

Keep in mind, not everyone in life will like you. That does not mean that you are not a likeable person. Do you like everyone that crosses your path? Of course not!

I like to use artwork as an example to demonstrate this concept. When you go to an art gallery, you have your opinions about which artwork you like and don't like. Maybe the person you are with likes a piece of art that you do not like. Preferences are based on opinions. Opinions are like bellybuttons – everyone has one. But the artwork does not change based on my opinion, or whether I favor it or disfavor it. Think of yourself as a piece of art! Who you are and your value as a person does not change based on the opinions of others.

Helpful Column

Let's reframe our belief and identify something more realistic.

Here is an example of a healthier way of thinking: *The person I saw at the store seemed a bit wrapped up in himself/herself. I wonder if there is something wrong? It's not personal. I am ok as a person. My value and worth does not depend on how others treat me or what others think of me.*

Nothing in this world is personal. Nothing. We all act from our own needs ALL OF THE TIME.

An amazing amount of freedom comes with the understanding that NOTHING IN THIS WORLD IS PERSONAL. The behaviors of others may *affect* us personally, but others do not do things to us because it is US. Their behavior is driven by who they are and what they need.

Now, let's return to our example. Considering the reframed perspective, how do I feel about the situation? Maybe now I feel *concerned* about the person since I am no longer taking the situation personally.

I no longer have a physiological response. I no longer feel a kick in the gut of rejection.

I also no longer need to avoid, but maybe instead *I call the person to make sure they are ok.* Observe how we tend to engage the world more frequently and more effectively when we frame our experiences more neutrally or positively.

Suppose I call the person and they say they didn't see me and apologize. Relationship saved! Furthermore, the longer I wait to make that call, the longer I suffer with my negative thoughts.

Suppose when I contact the person they tell me they actually saw me and they were, in fact, avoiding me because I talk too much. While this may seem hurtful, I don't need to take it personally. Maybe I do talk too much for that person, or maybe they are busy and don't have time to chat. Either way, it is not personal if someone does not want to chat. Remember, they are busy filling their own needs which have nothing to do with you.
Let's look at another example that involves anger.

ANGER EXAMPLE

Situation:	The cashier at the big box store is rude, rolls her eyes, throws my purchases in a bag, throws the receipt at me, won't make eye contact.	
	Unhelpful	**Helpful**
Thoughts: *(I am........)*	She is rude. I should not be treated this way. If I was important, I would not be treated this way. I'm not important. I don't matter.	I wonder if she is having a bad day. She is treating everyone badly. It's not personal. I'm ok. My value and worth does not depend on how others treat me.
Emotions/ Feelings	Angry	Concern, sympathy, empathy
Physical:	Increased heart rate, tense, hot face.	None, feel comfortable.
Action/Behavior:	Yell at her.	Tell her to have a good day and smile.

13

As you review this example, keep in mind that "anger management" courses teach people to breathe deeply, count to 10, and to think about the consequences of their anger.

In this situation, *I'm at the big box store and the cashier is rude, she is throwing my purchases in the plastic bags, throws the receipt at me, and won't make eye contact with me.*

My immediate interpretation of her behavior is that *she is rude and I should not be treated this way.*

Those thoughts may be true. But if I have a *"should"* in my thoughts, then I am setting myself up for disappointment because I am creating an expectation about how someone else should behave.

What does it mean about me that I "shouldn't" be treated this way? My core interpretation is that if I was important, like a VIP or a celebrity, the cashier would have treated me differently, which means that I am telling myself *that I am not important and I don't matter.*

These beliefs are open wounds just below the surface. They are luggage and baggage that I am carrying around from the past and every time I experience a situation like a rude cashier, it touches on those wounds which generates my emotional response of anger.

Often, in these situations, the anger bubbles to the surface very quickly. It happens so quickly that we don't realize there is a thought wedged in between the event and the emotion. Consequently, it deceptively appears that the cashier made me angry.

Someone or something cannot make you angry.

Anger comes from within.

Anger is a secondary emotion, which means that it is the reflection of another primary emotion, which is either hurt, fear, or frustration.

In the rude cashier example, the anger may be a reflection of all three primary emotions.

The hurt comes from the belief that I am not important and I don't matter.

The fear comes from what can happen if I am not considered important in this world. Important people get what they need in this world and I am at risk in some way by not being important.

The frustration comes from having my purchases squashed on top of each other and possibly damaged, as well as the frustration of not being able to control someone else's behavior.

The emotional response is accompanied by a physiological response of an *increased heart rate, becoming tense, getting hot face.* In this instance, my body is involuntarily preparing for the fight/flight response. The anger (fear) emotion is signaling my brain to prepare for the physical or psychological threat that my brain perceives in my environment.

The problem with anger is that the accompanying physiological response serves as a circular reinforcer of the emotion. The strong physical response reinforces the emotion and the emotion and interpretation of the situation generates the physical response.

My resulting behavior is to *yell at the cashier.* We have all seen (or maybe been) the person yelling at a cashier in anger. Now you know the chain of events that occurs when you witness someone upset with a cashier.

Helpful Column

Time to reframe that unhelpful thought again!

First, we obviously cannot control the cashier's behavior. We are going to encounter people in life who are rude. We are going to encounter people who do not treat us the way we "should" be treated, or treat us with respect. We can seek to *influence* the behavior of others, but we cannot control it.

What we can control is the way we think. Let's reframe the core belief we identified, "I am not important. I don't matter."

Remember, that belief is not true. If we think it is true, it is because we *FEEL* like it is true. But now you are learning that the way that we think determines how we feel.

A more helpful way to think about the situation of a rude cashier is *I wonder if she is having a bad day. She is treating everyone badly. It's not personal. I'm ok as a person. My value and worth does not depend on how others treat me.*

It doesn't even make sense that my value and worth would be dependent upon a cashier at a store who is a stranger to me. But if I get angry at a cashier, that belief is exactly what is being triggered in that situation. How can my value and worth be dependent upon how a stranger treats me? No wonder people walk around with anxiety!

Now what do I feel? *Concern, sympathy, and perhaps empathy.* I can genuinely empathize with the cashier because I am no longer taking the situation personally.

Notice now that I have no physiological response. There is no breathing deeply, counting to 10 or walking away. No anger management techniques are needed!

My resulting behavior is to *tell her to have a good day and smile at her.* There is no sarcasm, no gritting my words between my teeth, no snarky looks.

While the two examples provided may not apply to you, the concepts are the same. Many people do not struggle with anger or feelings of rejection but the cognitive process is the same.

For the blank worksheets, remember to identify the situation first, then identify your emotions using the word list provided, identify every word that applies, identify your thoughts using your emotional response as a guidepost, and then identify physical responses and finally, actions.

<u>Homework</u>

At this point, you may go to the HOMEWORK section and begin your homework for the day.

For further information and explanations about thoughts and beliefs, continue reading.

More about "Thoughts"

On average, 80% of our self-talk is negative. There are two main reasons for this phenomenon. First, negative cognitions (thoughts) and beliefs are created in childhood when there is little ability to challenge these thoughts and to understand the context and complexity of situations. Children have an inability to understand cause and effect. For example, if mom comes home and makes a comment about her bad day at work, then subsequently yells at the child out of frustration and exhaustion, the child will not make the connection between the cause (bad day at work) and the effect (yelling). Instead, what happens is the thought process, "mom is yelling because I did a bad thing. I am bad," is created. Extensive research exists that demonstrates the connection between verbal and emotional abuse in childhood and depression and anxiety in adulthood.

Second, retaining negative information is necessary for survival (our brain needs to be aware of potential or actual threats), while positive information is useless for survival purposes and is therefore discarded. The survival mechanisms in our brain are very powerful and generally work faster and overtake the thinking part of the brain. Negative information and experiences are stored in the neural pathways of the brain. So, if someone insults me and someone compliments me, who is more of a potential threat to me? Exactly – the one who insulted me. This mechanism is the reason the negative stays and the positive leaves. As we learn to be more aware of the positive, it becomes part of the neural structure rather than passing through.

"Just think positively!" has become almost cliché in our society but positive affirmations do play an important role in transforming lives. Positive thoughts create positive emotions which can actually affect our physiology. A concept called neuroplasticity, which is the brain's capacity to reorganize its structure and function, is a powerful tool that explains why positive affirmations work. The brain is malleable and we have the power and ability to generate positive change. However, because initial changes are temporary, it takes repetition and consistency to make changes permanent. Therefore, as we practice positive affirmations and gratitude, our brains strengthen those neural connections.

Each time our brain strengthens a connection, it simultaneously weakens a connection of neurons that weren't used in that moment. The brain can erase and override information that wasn't used, as it becomes irrelevant. Think about riding a mountain bike on a dirt trail. Imagine there are ruts on the trail into which the tire slips. With conscious effort, you can maneuver the bike to a different part of the trail. As you avoid the old rut and follow the new path, the old rut eventually fills in and disappears, while the new path will get deeper and the bike will begin to follow the new rut. The new rut becomes the automatic "go to." With practice, new thoughts can become our automatic "go to." New, positive thoughts can feel awkward and clunky at first but will eventually begin to feel normal.

Situation:	I'm at the big box store, walking down the aisle and someone I know walks by and does not acknowledge me.	
	Unhelpful	**Helpful**
Thoughts: *(I am.......)*	He/she ignored me. They don't like me. I am not likeable.	He/she looks a bit wrapped up in themselves. I wonder if there is something wrong? It's not personal. I'm ok. My value and worth does not depend on how others treat me or what others think of me.
Emotions/ Feelings	Low, sad, rejected	Concern
Physical:	Stomach cramps, low energy, feel sick	None, feel comfortable
Action/Behavior:	Go home and avoid them.	Get in touch and make sure they are ok.

Situation:	The cashier at the big box store is rude, rolls her eyes, throws my purchases in a bag, throws the receipt at me, won't make eye contact.	
	Unhelpful	**Helpful**
Thoughts: *(I am…….)*	She is rude. I should not be treated this way. If I was important, I would not be treated this way. I'm not important. I don't matter.	I wonder if she is having a bad day. She is treating everyone badly. It's not personal. I'm ok. My value and worth does not depend on how others treat me.
Emotions/ Feelings	Angry	Concern, sympathy, empathy
Physical:	Increased heart rate, tense, hot face.	None, feel comfortable.
Action/Behavior:	Yell at her.	Tell her to have a good day and smile.

	Unhelpful	Helpful
Situation:		
Thoughts: *(I am……..)*		
Emotions/ Feelings		
Physical:		
Action/Behavior:		

UNHELPFUL EMOTIONS/FEELINGS

ABANDONED	DESPAIR	INTIMIDATED	REPULSION
ABUSED	DETACHED	INVADED	RESENTFUL
ACCUSED	DISAPPOINTED	INVISIBLE	RESIGNED
AFRAID	DISCOURAGED	IRRITATED	REVULSION
ALIENATED	DISGUST	ISOLATED	RIDICULED
ALONE	DISTRUSTFUL	JEALOUS	SAD
ANGER	DOMINATED	JUDGED	SKEPTICAL
ANIMOSITY	EMBARRASED	LONELY	SMOTHERED
ANNOYED	EMPTY	LOST	SORROW
ANXIOUS	FEAR	MAD	SORRY
ASHAMED	FEARFUL	MANIPULATED	SUFFOCATED
ATTACKED	FOOLISH	MISERABLE	SUSPICIOUS
BELITTLED	FRUSTRATED	MISLED	TENSE
BETRAYED	GUILTY	MISTREATED	TERRIFIED
BLAMED	GUTLESS	MISUNDERSTOOD	THREATENED
BORED	HATE	MOCKED	TIMID
CHEATED	HELPLESS	MORTIFIED	TRAPPED
COLD	HOPELESS	NEGLECTED	UNAPPRECIATED
CONFUSED	HUMILIATED	NERVOUS	UNEASY
CONTROLLED	HURT	NUMB	UNHEARD
CORNERED	IGNORED	OBLIGATED	UNIMPORTANT
COWARDLY	IMPRISONED	OFFENDED	UNLOVED
CRUSHED	INADEQUATE	PARALYZED	UNSAFE
DAMAGED	INCAPABLE	PATHETIC	UNSUPPORTED
DEFENSELESS	INDIFFERENT	POWERLESS	USED
DEFENSIVE	INDIGNATION	PRESSURED	USELESS
DEGRADED	INFURIATED	PUNISHED	VIOLATED
DEHUMANIZED	INFERIOR	REJECTED	VULNERABLE
DEPRESSED	INSECURE	REMORSEFUL	WITHDRAWN
DEPRIVED	INSIGNIFICANT	REPELLED	WORTHLESS

HOMEWORK DAY 1

QUOTE OF THE DAY:

*OWNING YOUR OWN FEELINGS, RATHER THAN BLAMING THEM ON
SOMEONE ELSE, IS THE MARK OF A PERSON WHO HAS MOVED FROM
CONTRACTED TO EXPANDED AWARENESS. – DEEPAK CHOPRA*

1) Complete 3 ABC worksheets using the following types of situations:

- A painful event from childhood. It can involve parents, family, school, bullying, abuse, etc.
- An event relating to an intimate relationship, past or present.
- An event that occurred today.

2) Make a commitment to complete Day 2.

GOOD JOB TODAY! I KNOW YOU CAN DO IT!!!

DAY 2 BOUNDARIES

Today's Objective: 1) Learn what boundaries are 2) Learn how to set and maintain boundaries 3) Begin to eliminate unhealthy boundaries 4) Begin implementing healthy boundaries in your life

The topic of boundaries is vast, but for Boot Camp purposes, we will approach boundaries from an introductory perspective and begin with a basic outline of the concepts that embody *boundaries*. For more information on boundaries, there are many excellent books and workbooks on the market that provide more detail.

Boundaries are incredibly important when it comes to mental health. Unhealthy boundaries play a significant role in depression and anxiety symptoms.

For those with unhealthy boundaries, establishing healthy ones will be a monumental undertaking. Establishing healthy boundaries involves multiple steps which include: learning what boundaries are; identifying where unhealthy boundaries exist; improving self-esteem while identifying the right within yourself assert healthy boundaries; practicing new and healthy boundaries in small ways; practicing new healthy boundaries in important areas and relationships; dealing with push back (people who are accustomed to violating your boundaries will wish to continue to do so); and continually exerting your right to new boundaries and recovering from relapses.

Let's begin by defining boundaries. Consider boundaries as an invisible line in human interactions, whether physical or psychological, that defines acceptable parameters. When crossed, the boundary violation generates an emotional response and damages the person, persons, and/or the relationship.

The easiest, more classic example of a boundary is a property line. Property lines define what is and is not my property. If someone decides to bring their belongings and set up a yard sale on my property, I have the right to tell them to leave my property. Psychological boundaries are no different. Psychological boundaries include mental, emotional, and spiritual boundaries. Physical boundaries include material and bodily boundaries.

It is important to understand some basic concepts. Boundaries are not ultimatums. Ultimatums are threats, coercions, or manipulations. When beginning to implement new boundaries, many people often mistakenly resort to issuing ultimatums. If you look at boundaries as more of an exchange or offering of information in order to create understanding, you are more likely to be successful with boundary implementation.

For example, rather than saying "Don't talk to me that way," which connotes an underlying threat, a healthier way of asserting your emotional/verbal, emotional boundary would be "When you tell me that my idea to write a book is stupid, it hurts my feelings. I would prefer words of encouragement instead." We will further discuss how to communicate effectively on Day 9, Healthy Communication.

Another falsehood about boundaries is that "No" embodies the totality of the message you need to communicate. If you recall, establishing healthy boundaries involves creating understanding. A simple "No" is not likely to create understanding and may be perceived as hostility. That said, there may be times when "No" is appropriate. Remember, creating understanding is about connectivity; hostility is about separation. Most of the time we (as humans) desire connectivity; sometimes we need separation. Below are some examples of when using "No" alone may be interpreted with an unintended hostile undertone.

Do you want to discuss our disagreement? No.

A better response that conveys a different, more understanding attitude would be:

Do you want to discuss our disagreement? No, I'm not ready yet. But I will come to you soon when I am ready to talk.

Just a small explanation eliminates a potential misinterpretation of hostility and fosters understanding.

Here is another example:

Would you be available to help me on Saturday? No.

Again, simply saying "No" may leave room for misinterpretation. A better alternative might be:

Would you be available to help me on Saturday? No, I have to work. Is there another day I could help for a couple hours?

The response with an explanation asserts a healthier boundary because it establishes what I am willing to offer, when, and for how long. It also sidetracks unintended consequences such as perceived hostility. After all, hostility is (generally) a violation of someone else's boundary.

This concept is especially important when it comes to electronic communication, such as text messages and email. When tone of voice and intonations are not conveyed, opportunities for misinterpretation abound.

Defining Physical Boundaries

Physical boundaries include material and bodily boundaries, encompassing my physical body and the space immediately surrounding it.

Material boundaries include property (such as your home), personal belongings (such as your vehicle), personal items (such as clothes and home furnishings), and your services and/or labor (such as helping with tasks). An example might include friends asking to borrow your pick-up truck and returning it dirty, damaged, or empty. Another example may include friends or family expecting your tax accounting services for free.

Bodily boundaries relate to your physical body and your personal space. Notice how uncomfortable you feel when you encounter a "close talker." Bodily boundaries include who can touch you, how they can touch you, where they can touch you, and when they can touch you. Bodily boundaries also include sexual boundaries. An example of bodily boundaries would be a boss who routinely touches or hugs a subordinate without permission.

Psychological Boundaries

Psychological boundaries include mental, emotional, and spiritual boundaries.

Mental boundaries include thoughts, values, opinions, and beliefs. An example would include imposing your own values or beliefs on another person, such as "You should teach your kids about the importance of volunteering in the community." Volunteering may be an important value in my family, but that may not be the case in someone else's family.

Emotional boundaries are about separating your feelings from someone else's in a healthy way. While the basis of human connection is emotional bonding, and empathy is an important skill, you are entitled to your own feelings and you do not have to assume the burden of other people's feelings. Healthy emotional boundaries include knowing where you end and I begin, being your own person, being aware of your own feelings (and your right to have them), being aware of the impact of your behavior on the feelings of others. There is a difference between feeling responsible for the emotional well-being of others and owning the emotional impact your behavior has on others.

An example would include giving feedback to someone about an idea they presented. If the other person's feelings were hurt by your comments, they have a responsibility to let you know and you have a responsibility to apologize and make amends. If the person comes to you and tells you that it is your fault that they lost the confidence to pursue their idea - that is not your responsibility. They are responsible for managing their own emotions and behaviors. We will discuss how to effectively heal hurts on Day 20. Suffice to say, sometimes "I'm sorry" isn't enough!

Spiritual boundaries relate to the spiritual aspect of our beliefs. For some people, spiritual boundaries include organized religion. For others, spirituality may involve less formal forms of beliefs, such as attunement with nature or the universe. Discussing spirituality is not necessarily a boundary violation but disparaging or discounting another person's religion is a violation.

Identifying Boundaries

Some questions to consider when beginning the process of identifying boundaries:

Am I having an emotional response in this situation?

If so, what am I feeling? (Use the word list from Day 1 and do an ABC worksheet if needed.)

What type of boundary was violated?

What type of boundary did I violate in someone else?

What do I find offensive?

Who seems to be a source of unhealthy boundaries in my life?

To further identify your personal boundaries, complete the following assessment:

PERSONAL BOUNDARY ASSESSMENT

	Not at all 1	Not often 2	Sometimes 3	All the time 4
I have a difficult time saying no to people				
If I say no to someone in my personal life, I feel guilty				
If I say no to someone at work, I feel guilty				
If I say no to someone in my family, I feel guilty				
I easily have my feelings hurt				
I am afraid of falling apart				
If someone hurts my feelings, I have difficulty telling them.				
I would describe myself as a doormat				
Others describe me as a doormat				
I would describe myself as aggressive towards others				
Others would describe me as aggressive towards others				
I care what other people think				
I try not to have opinions about things				
I am not tolerant of other points of view				
I am not tolerant of other religions				
I need to know what is going on in other people's lives				
I need to 'be in the know' at work				
I don't trust people easily or at all				
I put the needs and wants of others before my own				
I try to fix the problems of others				
I need to control other people				
Other people would describe me as controlling				
I need to control situations				
I allow others to determine how I spend my time				
I avoid conflict then feel resentful				
I expect reciprocal treatment for my time or generosity				
I expect loyalty for giving my own loyalty				
I often use anger or intimidation to get my way				
I often allow others to violate my personal space against my wishes				
I have a difficult time expressing my emotions				

I find myself stressed and overwhelmed frequently				
I feel like other people run my life (kids, spouse, parents, friends, boss)				
I allow others to take advantage of me				
I hate disappointing people and avoid it				
I get upset if someone doesn't like me				
If someone criticizes me, I believe it and fall apart				
I let others define me				
I am afraid to question or challenge professionals even when I am paying for their service (doctors, lawyers, accountants, auto repair)				

If your scores are mostly 3s and 4s, there are some unhealthy boundaries at play in your life.

Now that we have identified what boundaries are and conducted a preliminary assessment of your personal boundaries, let's further identify the functioning of boundaries in various areas of your life with the following worksheet:

BOUNDARY INVENTORY

For each area, assess the overall functioning in the relationship. Consider whether you see areas that need improvement. Ask yourself if there are times when you feel uncomfortable, if you feel people pulling away, if you find people avoiding you, how far off are these relationships from where you want them to be, what does an ideal relationship in this area look like, and what prevents an ideal relationship from existing. You may need an additional piece of paper to address all aspects of the boundaries within each category.

MARRIAGE/INTIMATE RELATIONSHIP:

PARENTS:

CHILDREN:

SIBLINGS:

OTHER FAMILY MEMBERS:

FRIENDS:

WORK/COWORKERS/SCHOOL:

THE GENERAL PUBLIC/OTHERS:

<u>Establishing Boundaries</u>

Using the information you identified on the previous worksheet, identify who violates your boundaries and why.

Begin having your boundaries heard and understood with those who violate your boundaries. Often, the same person exhibits the same pattern in the same categories and may exhibit the pattern with others, as well. Ask yourself why this person finds their behavior acceptable, think about whether or not they are aware of their boundary crossing, and if it is malicious. If your boundaries are violated by multiple people in the same category, you will need to begin to address the issue first within yourself, then with others.

Watch what happens in your life when you begin to establish healthy boundaries with others. Often, those closest to you will not like the new you, but they will eventually come to accept it.

When setting boundaries, consider:

Am I easily offended? Am I being sensible and rational? (Hint: ABC worksheets are an extremely effective way to discover how you are interpreting situations to determine if you are overly sensitive.)

Remember, boundaries are not about issuing ultimatums or shutting people out. They are intended to improve relationships and interactions.

Not everyone is familiar with the concept of boundaries. However, by establishing your own, you can control your own emotional well-being and positively influence your relationships with others without waiting for them to change.

Boundaries are assertive, not aggressive. We will discuss this concept further on Day 9, Healthy Communication. Often people don't realize their communication is aggressive. It's not what you say, it's how you say it. Being assertive is about standing up FOR yourself. Being aggressive is standing AGAINST someone else. Being aggressive cuts you off from others, as they will distance themselves in order to avoid having their boundaries violated. When we feel violated, it is natural to instinctively aggress against someone else, but the purpose of boundaries is to foster healthy connectivity. Stronger relationships cannot happen when communication is peppered with aggressive overtures.

Setting healthy boundaries does not include making up excuses or white lies. Be calm, matter-of-fact, polite, and confident. Stick to the point. Do not allow others to use distraction or minimization techniques. And do not get talked out of your boundaries – or your right to them.

Keys to Setting Boundaries

Remember, the main idea with setting boundaries is to convey information and create understanding.

The most effective method for setting boundaries is to state your boundary with the preferred alternative. Use the framework of acknowledging the existing behavior and identifying or requesting the preferred behavior.

Here is the format:

I know you're accustomed to (behavior), but I would prefer it if you would (behavior).

In the earlier example of a physically touch-friendly boss, establishing a healthy boundary would look like this:

"I know you are a hugger but I'm more comfortable with a handshake than a hug."

Other examples of healthy boundary language include:

You can ask someone, "Is there anything I can do for you? I am available to listen. Do you want my help? Do you want any suggestions? What is it that you need?"

You can state, "I have a concern. May I share it with you?"

If someone asks you, "What should I do, or what would you do?" your reply might be: "I can share with you what I might do in that situation" or "What do you think are your options?"

You can tell someone, "I cannot participate in this conversation. This interaction is not healthy for you or me. This interaction is pushing me away from you." You always have the option of leaving, especially if there is an escalation in the conversation.

You can keep someone on topic by stating, "We can talk about your concern/issue but first I would like to finish addressing the issue I brought up."

Boundary Practice

As you begin to incorporate new boundaries, recognize that, just like any other skill, you will need to practice, you will make mistakes, you will have a learning curve, and it will become easier and more natural with continued practice.

Expect challenges to your newly established boundaries. You may not be taken seriously at first, so others may continue their existing/offending behaviors, and new boundaries may need to be reasserted. Make sure you are consistent with new boundaries in order to create change. Change doesn't happen overnight but consistency will lend to the process.

Use the following My Boundaries with Others worksheet as a guide for identifying unhealthy boundaries and establishing new boundaries.

MY BOUNDARIES WITH OTHERS

SITUATION/ WHAT I SAID OR DID	MY INTERPRETATION OF SITUATION	HOW I FELT	UNHEALTHY BOUNDARY	NEW BOUNDARY (try using "I know you're accustomed to...but I would prefer...)
EXAMPLE: My child did not do her chores, went to basketball game with her friends after being told no.	I am a horrible parent and cannot even control my own child. She does not respect me. I am not worthy of respect.	Disrespected Powerless Unloved Inadequate	Yelled at her, punished her, took her car away.	Have a talk with her calmly. Discuss consequences of her choices and set up a parenting consequence chart to teach her rather than punish her. "I know you are accustomed to disobeying me instead of following instructions but I would prefer that you listen when I tell you no."
EXAMPLE: My husband tells our friends what a terrible cook I am.	I am a bad wife. I am incompetent.	Disrespected Unloved Incompetent Embarrassed	I ignore it and try to laugh it off. I don't address his hurtful statements with him.	Talk to him. "I know you are accustomed to teasing me in front of others about my cooking but I would prefer less teasing and more positive comments about me to others."
EXAMPLE: My coworker does not do his fair share of work and often stands around while others pick up the slack.	I have to get the work done and don't have the right to speak up. Speaking up will just cause problems.	Burdened Obligated Used Disrespected	Ignore the situation and do the extra work.	Address the issue. "I know you are used to the rest of us making sure all of the work gets done but I would prefer if you would pitch in more and help us make sure all of the clients are contacted."
EXAMPLE: My friend constantly runs late when we meet for lunch.	She doesn't respect me. I am not worthy of respect. She doesn't care about my time or our friendship.	Offended Frustrated Unworthy	Show up late for lunch. Stop meeting her for lunch. Back away from the friendship.	Address the issue with her. "I know you are accustomed to running late when we meet for lunch but I would prefer if you could meet on time instead of having me wait 15 minutes for you."

MY BOUNDARIES WITH OTHERS

SITUATION/ WHAT I SAID OR DID	MY INTERPRETATION OF SITUATION	HOW I FELT	UNHEALTHY BOUNDARY	NEW BOUNDARY (try using "I know you're accustomed to...but I would prefer...)

HOMEWORK DAY 2

1) Complete a "My Boundaries With Others" worksheet with at least 3 examples of unhealthy boundaries in your life. It is helpful to use different areas of your life such as family, intimate relationships, casual relationships, friendships, work, or strangers in public.

2) Complete an ABC worksheet on any situation.

3) Make a commitment to complete Day 3.

I KNOW YOU CAN DO IT!!!

DAY 3 THE FIVE PSYCHOLOGICAL FEARS

Today's Objective: 1) Learn about the five categories of psychological fears 2) Learn how they impact and influence your behaviors 3) Begin to challenge your fears

When we think of the word fear, we usually think of being afraid of a thing like monsters, bad guys, crimes, being hurt physically. But we can also be afraid of things that don't physically exist, namely, emotional pain.

The part of the brain that registers physical fear is the same part of the brain that registers psychological fear. Our psychological fears can be significant behavioral motivators. If we are aware of our psychological fears, we have a greater ability to control and manage them and our resulting behaviors.

In today's lesson, we will learn about five categories of psychological fears and use a worksheet to begin to address our fears.

There are five categories of psychological fear; extinction, mutilation, loss of autonomy, separation, and ego-death. The last two fear categories are the biggest drivers of human behavior.

Fear of Extinction

The fear of extinction is the fear of ceasing to exist; it is beyond the fear of death. It is the existential fear of no longer existing in any form.

Intellectually, we are all aware of ultimate death. We are terminal creatures and none of us will live eternally. Our lives have an end date. Most of us assume we will live to old age.

For various reasons, this fear is more pronounced for some people. For those who have witnessed death, experienced a near-death event, or lost a loved one, death is conceptually more real than intellectual.

Examples of the fear of extinction include fear of heights, fear of falling, and fear of bridges. The fear of heights isn't about the height, it is the prospect that a fall from that height will cause my death and I will cease to exist.

Fear of Mutilation

The fear of mutilation is a fear of the loss of: part of our body, use of part of our body, or mutilation of part of our body. This fear extends beyond contemplation of the initial physical pain. The physical pain associated with mutilation usually ends, so part of our fear is associated with the resulting impact of the injury.

Examples of fear of mutilation include a fear of bugs, spiders, snakes, and other animals. Most spiders, especially household spiders, are not harmful and don't bite. And yet, when many people see spiders, they have visions of the spider jumping on them, crawling all over them, losing sight of it, and finally being bitten.

Fear of heights can also be included in this category. If I start climbing a ladder, I may begin getting nervous, most likely with visions of a broken leg or neck and the loss of the use of parts of my body either temporarily or permanently. The higher I climb, my fear converts to fear of extinction when the consequences of a fall could be fatal.

Fear of extinction and mutilation generally have little day to day impact on our lives. However, for some it can impact daily functioning.

One of the easiest ways of tackling fears in these two categories is the use of cognitively challenging the statistical probability of the fear. What that means is asking yourself, "What are the chances of this happening?"

For people with previous negative experiences, the instinctive, survival mechanisms in the brain can generate a powerful fear response. For example, a person who was bitten by a dog as a child may develop an intense fear of dogs.

A great example of using statistics to cognitively challenge fears involves the fear of flying. Many people are afraid of flying on an airplane, yet more people are injured or killed in auto accidents than plane crashes. Statistically, millions of people fly safely every year.

Two dynamics contribute to the fear of flying. For those have this fear, the emotional response itself unknowingly confirms the belief that flying is dangerous. We assume, "If I feel afraid, I must be in danger."

But, based on our lesson on Day 1, now you know that the fearful feelings, in the absence of actual danger, come from our thoughts, not from the situation. Now we know to challenge our thoughts to lessen our emotional response. Our new thought might be, "The chances of dying on this flight are almost zero."

The second dynamic at play in fueling our fears is overgeneralization. When a plane crashes, we are inundated with news coverage of the event. When our brain witnesses these images, it registers the event as more prevalent than it actually is. Naturally, we don't see all of the flights that occur safely every day, so we subconsciously link the crash event to flights, generally.

News outlets notoriously report and sensationalize negative events. The images and stories we see contribute to our depression and anxiety. Turn off the news for a week and see what happens to your overall well-being!

To further resolve fear of extinction and mutilation, we will introduce specific exercises on Day 11, Anxiety, to address those fears.

Fear of Loss of Autonomy

The fear of loss of autonomy involves the fear of being immobilized, trapped, restricted, enveloped, overwhelmed, smothered, or controlled by circumstances. This fear surfaces in various situations, but mostly in the context of relationships. Many people have a fear of commitment to relationships. The fear is not in the commitment itself, but in the fear that the commitment represents being trapped or stuck in the relationship.

Think of an anxious bride or groom. The fear about getting married is not the marriage itself; it is the fear that the relationship will sour and they will feel trapped in the marriage. The trapped aspect of the relationship is not being physically trapped, but being situationally trapped.

Fear of Separation

The fear of separation involves the fear of abandonment, rejection, losing connectedness with others; being seen as a non-person, being unwanted, disrespected, or not valued by anyone else.

One example of the fear of separation involves our reaction when we are the recipient of the silent treatment. If my partner is angry with me and won't speak to me, it may arouse fear and anxiety, which stems from the fear of being rejected and losing connectedness with that person. Adults who use the silent treatment towards children can arouse a very intense fear of abandonment in the child, thus possibly planting the seeds of anxiety and also contributing to the development of abandonment issues.

Another example of fear of separation involves the emotion of jealousy. Jealousy represents the fear of being perceived as less valuable, that others will be seen as more valuable than I am, and being abandoned in favor of others who are more valuable. Think about the hatred spewed toward celebrities at times; it often originates from jealousy because of their perceived value due to their wealthy and privileged lifestyles.

Ego-Death

This fear is a major driver of behavior. Ego-death involves the fear of humiliation, shame, or any other form of disapproval that damages a person's ego, which is the constructed sense of self – essentially, who we are. Ego-death is the shattering or injury to a person's sense of lovability, competence, or worth.

Examples of this fear include fear of rejection, such as a guy being nervous about approaching a cute girl. The guy must put his ego on the line to speak to her and risk possible rejection. Think about how many times people have avoided approaching someone to dodge the potential sting of rejection.

I know what you're thinking and it shows tremendous progress. The guy should do an ABC worksheet, realize the rejection isn't personal, and generate a "Helpful" column that includes talking to the girl!!!

Another example of ego-death is the fear of public speaking. Why are people so afraid and anxious about public speaking? At the core of the fear of public speaking is having to face humiliation if the speech/presentation goes poorly or if someone asks a question you can't answer. The feeling of humiliation stems from having to endure the ego hit of being incapable.

The purpose of understanding the five psychological fears is to be able to identify where these various fears show up in your life. It is much easier to challenge and resolve fears (and resulting behaviors) if you can identify them.

Use the following worksheet to identify a situation or example of when you feel nervous, anxious, or fearful. In the next column, identify a category of fears or a specific fear using the suggested list. In the third column, titled "Obstacle," identify an obstacle you put in your way to avoid feeling your fear. In the last column, see if you can identify one step you can take to remove the obstacle and confront your fear.

LIST OF FEARS

Intimacy

Disconnection

Rejection

Failure

Disapproval

Being Judged

Making a Mistake

Change

Being Trapped

Loss of Freedom

Being Smothered

The Unknown

Being Invisible

Disappointment

Pain

Illness

Being Controlled

Being Out of Control

Dominated

Abandonment

Being a Victim

Inadequacy

Death

Humiliation

Devalued

Excluded

Loneliness

Ridicule

Ostracized

Suppression

Being Used

Being Guilted

Shame

Being Ignored

Being Neglected

Being Unheard

OVERCOMING MY FEARS			
EXAMPLES			
SITUATION	**FEAR**	**OBSTACLE**	**STEP**
I'm always single. I date people for a few weeks at a time.	Loss of Autonomy Dominated Loss of Control	Avoiding relationships.	Go on a date and refrain from finding minor things wrong with the person.
Driving out of my way to avoid going over a bridge.	Extinction	Won't drive over bridges, drive out of my way, sometimes drive up to three hours out of my way.	Use cognitive techniques to challenge fear.
Relationships never work out. I date needy people and end up resenting them.	Fear of Separation Abandonment	Dating someone who is poor who I must take care of so they will need me.	Do ABC worksheet and realize why I keep dating people who are "safe" choices/needy. Do analysis of how past relationships have ended.
Avoid getting my masters because I know the program requires being video-taped.	Ego-Death	Don't finish my masters. Stuck in my job and can't move up.	Do ABC worksheet, challenge my fear of being video-taped. Video tape myself and watch it.
Staying in a bad relationship.	Fear of Separation Alone Disconnected	Ignore the problems in the relationship. Justify problems. Make excuses.	Recognize why I ignore and justify issues in the relationship.
My kids want me to go skydiving with them.	Extinction Death	Avoid going skydiving.	Look at statistics and safety of skydiving.
Social anxiety about going places that are new or going alone.	Ego Death Judged	I avoid doing things alone or wait until others can go with me.	Recognize my fear is about being judged by others.
My partner comments that I don't open up to him.	Loss of Autonomy Fear of Separation Ego-Death	I don't open up to partners in relationships.	Recognize my fears, recognize what I have to lose by not being open and vulnerable, begin with small disclosures about myself.
I want to leave my job but don't have confidence to apply for jobs.	Ego-Death Rejection Failure	I don't apply for jobs, stuck and unhappy in my job.	Recognize my lack of confidence is about doubts about my capabilities, fear of being rejected and not being good enough. Apply for job, practice interview skills.

OVERCOMING MY FEARS

SITUATION	FEAR	OBSTACLE	STEP
Identify a situation in your life where you feel nervous, anxious, fear; areas of your life that are problematic or where there is inaction.	*Look at the list of fears and identify a specific fear or category of fears.*	*What obstacles do you put in your way to avoid feeling and confronting your fear? (Ex. Drinking, shutting down, working, isolating.)*	*Identify one step you can take to remove an obstacle.*

HOMEWORK DAY 3

1) Complete Overcoming My Fears worksheet. Begin to implement a behavior identified in the "Step" column.

2) Complete an ABC worksheet on any situation.

3) Make a commitment to complete Day 4.

YOU'VE GOT THIS!!!

DAY 4 DEFENSE MECHANISMS

Today's Objective: 1) Learn about the concept of defense mechanisms 2) Learn how they impact emotions and behavior 3) Learn how to identify them 4) Begin to challenge and change unhealthy defense mechanisms for improved functioning

Extensive literature exists about the ego and defense mechanisms. It is an important concept to touch on in order to understand the motivation for some of our functioning. Simply put, a defense mechanism is something we do to psychologically protect ourselves. Most people are unaware that they are using a defense mechanism that may be fueling depression and anxiety. Frequently, these behaviors begin in childhood and will continue if they work for us in some way.

Defense mechanisms range from basic/simple to complex. A classic example of a basic defense mechanism is denial. If I break a toy as a child, my parents asks if I did it, I respond 'no,' they believe me, nothing bad happens, and they buy me a new toy, I will learn very quickly that denial works and it works well. Alternatively, if I do not get a new toy, I will learn that the denial worked, but not as well as the first scenario. If my parent confronts me with the broken toy in my hand and addresses the denial in a healthy way (telling me that it is not ok to lie and assigning an appropriate consequence), I will learn that denial doesn't work. However, denial may play a role in my survival if my caregiver is physically abusive. My defense mechanisms may serve a life or death purpose. If denial helps me escape harm from a physically abusive caregiver, these defense mechanisms are strongly reinforced in the brain.

What may work in childhood may not work in adulthood. Denial as a survival mechanism in childhood may turn into lying behaviors in adulthood. When denying the truth proves effective, altering the truth may later become convenient. These behaviors often become sources of depression and anxiety.

As part of your journey to release those unhealthy beliefs and move toward the best version of you, let's explore some of the defense mechanisms individuals use, then we will use a worksheet to further assist with changing these dynamics.

Denial (basic): Denial is the refusal to accept reality as presented or experienced because the resulting consequence would be psychologically painful. Denial is used to avoid feelings, people, or situations. In addition to the above example, a person who denies having an alcohol problem may not want to face or confront the dynamics that underlie the drinking behaviors and will use denial or minimizing to avoid addressing the issue. Denial circumvents the need for change.

Regression (basic): Regression involves reverting to an earlier developmental stage. An example of regression is baby talking in adult relationships. If I am discussing something with my partner that I find uncomfortable, and talking like a baby works to "smooth over" my upset partner, I will become reliant upon this behavior to get me out of "trouble" or get me out of having to discuss something I want to avoid. This dynamic fuels anxiety in that I may subconsciously worry that the baby talk will not work someday or will not work for a bigger issue and I will be left to face an unpleasant or painful situation without any defenses or protection.

44

Acting out (basic): A child throwing a temper tantrum is a classic example of an acting out defense mechanism. An adult male equivalent is a 'mantrum.' (Women have tantrums, too!) As a child, it may work for me to get my way, such as crying to avoid eating my dinner, or throwing a toy to protest putting the toys away. In adulthood, acting out becomes an unhealthy way of managing not getting our way.

Dissociation (basic): We all dissociate in mild forms – losing track of time or daydreaming. For abuse survivors, dissociating, or disconnecting from the real world or finding a different representation of themselves can become a survival mechanism. Dissociating is the mind's way of protecting itself in the face of something psychologically overwhelming. It makes sense that when experiencing horrific abuse, the mind would go elsewhere. After the abuse ends, it is common for people to continue to dissociate due to an intolerance for overwhelming memories, emotions, or situations.

Compartmentalization (basic): When people mentally section parts of themselves off, it becomes a way of shielding the self from undesirable behaviors. If I perform an undesirable behavior, such as stealing, I can still refer to myself as a good person if I section off that behavior. Compartmentalizing keeps us from making progress and keeps us from examining those parts of ourselves that may need improvement.

Projection (basic): Projection is imposing on others what we dislike and cannot face in ourselves. By projecting, it removes what is undesirable in us and places the responsibility to address it on someone else. For example, a person with a lot of struggles and mental health issues may tell others that they need to seek help for their problems.

Repression (moderate): Repression is the blocking or squashing down of unpleasant thoughts and emotions and is often done unconsciously. It is the mind's natural urge to push away unwanted and painful thoughts and feelings. Trauma survivors often use repression for unprocessed memories. Our brains are designed to continually process events, information, and emotions. Much like breathing, it is an involuntary response. Processing is the mechanism for converting information from short term to long term memory. During traumatic events, this mechanism stops in order for the systems necessary to keep us alive to function at optimum capacity. The lack of processing of events may work well for survival, but results in an unprocessed memory getting stuck in short term memory. As this information tumbles around in our minds in a chaotic fashion, our natural inclination is to push away, or avoid, the painful memories and the painful emotions associated with it. Unfortunately, avoidance works very temporarily but results in the unprocessed information fueling depression and anxiety.

Displacement (moderate): Similar to projection, displacement involves directing unpleasant emotions onto someone or something. An example is making a mistake at work, getting in trouble by the boss, then kicking the dog later at home. The displacement involves an inability to accept making a mistake.

Rationalization (moderate): Rationalizing involves making excuses in order to avoid having to accept fault. This defense mechanism protects the self by blaming others or by blaming a situation. For example, I may rationalize overspending by telling myself that "I deserve it" or rationalize getting dumped by telling myself that the person was crazy or a loser and I didn't want that person anyway.

Compensation (complex): A way of avoiding facing and confronting my weaknesses is to counterbalance a weakness with a strength, thereby avoiding having to face or accept the weakness, such as excusing being a bad husband by being a good financial provider. By focusing on being a good provider, the other areas are not addressed and result in poor relationship outcomes. However, when compensation is used to reinforce positive qualities, it can be a healthy way to reinforce self-esteem. For example, if I focus on the fact that I am a good, loving mother but not the best cook, this approach serves to boost my self-esteem and avoid self-condemnation that fuel depression and anxiety. The weaknesses are not avoided, but rather accepted and incorporated as part of who I am.

Use the following worksheet to identify and challenge unhealthy defense mechanisms.

DEFENSE MECHANISMS WORKSHEET

SITUATION	DEFENSE MECHANISM (Denial, Acting Out, Dissociation, Compartmentalization, Projection, Repression, Displacement, Rationalization, Compensation)	WHERE DID THIS COME FROM?	WHAT AM I AVOIDING?	HOW COULD I HANDLE THE ISSUE WITHOUT A DEFENSE MECHANISM?
Example: I yelled at my kids.	*Acting Out Projection Displacement*	*I learned yelling from my mother. My husband is unhappy in our marriage. I hate my job, it is soul-sucking and I am afraid to change careers.*	*I feel incompetent as a mother. I feel out of control. I can't get them to behave or listen. I project onto them not being perfect. I am frustrated with my life, marriage, and job.*	*Get parenting help and marriage counseling. Focus on giving them a good childhood. Think about how they experience me as a mother. Recognize that it is ok to not be perfect. View parenting as teaching and they are in the process of learning and will make mistakes.*

HOMEWORK DAY 4

1) Complete Defense Mechanisms worksheet. Practice handling a situation where you do not utilize a defense mechanism.

2) Complete an ABC worksheet on any situation.

3) Make a commitment to complete Day 5.

KEEP YOUR COMMITMENT GOING!!!

DAY 5 CHILDHOOD ABUSE

Today's Objective: 1) Learn about the impact of all types of childhood abuse on adult functioning 2) Learn why adults often can't just "get over it" 3) Begin to explore the role abuse plays in our self-image 4) Begin the journey of creating a new, healthy belief system

"Childhood creates the filter through which we view the world." – Kristin Stonesifer, LCSW.

The topic of childhood abuse is vast and complex. For purposes of this book, we will examine the impact of all types of childhood abuse on functioning and mental health.

Construction of the Belief System

Every individual has a set of core beliefs that comprise his/her constructed sense of self. Everyone has a way of viewing who they are *as a person*. This self-image, or constructed sense of self, is the product of a combination of genetics, biology, and principally the product of early childhood experiences. In particular, healthy attachment and attunement from our primary caregivers has a profound effect on the construction of who we are and how we view ourselves.

Every experience we have as a child has an impact on who we are. The actions of our caregivers teach us about love, relationships, trust, the safety of the world, what we believe to be true about who we are, and what we believe about our value and our importance. Every experience becomes part of our inner working model of how the world works and how we function in it. Babies and children who have attuned caregivers (caregivers who react consistently and reliably to the child's emotional and physical needs) learn that others and the world are safe, predictable, trustworthy, and that the child herself has importance and therefore, inherent value.

If attunement and healthy attachment are crucial to the healthy emotional and physical development of a child, then what happens when children experience a caregiver who is not attuned? What happens to a child who experiences a caregiver who is not attuned and also abusive in some way? Not surprisingly, often this constellation of parental behaviors occurs together.

Abuse and the Belief System

For children raised by caregivers who are not attuned and who perpetrate abuse, a variety of factors contribute to a wide range of outcomes. Interestingly, these outcomes may not correlate to the level of abuse experienced. Survivors of satanic ritual abuse may function quite well while the child of divorce may struggle with anxiety and depression. For children who are abused, the messages that are directly and indirectly sent to the child are negative, which have a damaging impact on the child's developing belief system.

Think about a baby that is repeatedly left crying in her crib for extended periods of time who is hungry and has a dirty diaper. She will eventually learn to adapt to her environment and she will learn that she cannot trust anyone else to meet her needs. Her adaptations will include refraining from expressing her needs and also suppressing them. She will learn to rely only on herself and avoid trusting or relying on others. Even a baby who cannot consciously reason will begin to develop a specific, negative belief system. Young children are egocentric in that they only understand the world as it relates to them. With this simplistic model of the world, whatever happens to them is bad because of them. They lack the ability to reason beyond themselves and this misunderstanding forms the basis of a belief system that will be the foundation upon which they build their sense of self.

Beliefs that are common for abuse survivors include "I don't matter" or "I'm not as good as other people" or "I am unlovable." These beliefs are created during (and generated by) the course of abuse and neglect. For example, a child who is ignored when they look up from building a tower of blocks in search of approval will learn "What I'm doing doesn't matter; therefore, I don't matter." These experiences that are paired with a negative message form the foundation of our belief system. Going forward, we accept and incorporate examples that confirm our existing beliefs, thus strengthening them, and we reject examples that challenge or contradict our negative beliefs.

Consequently, abuse is damaging to our foundational belief system. This system underlies the manner in which we engage the world. Our core belief system is key in contributing to our emotional responses and our behavioral repertoire. For example, if I have a core belief that I am unlovable because I am overweight, I will probably feel sad, depressed, undesirable, and worthless. This pattern will probably contribute to sabotaging or avoiding behaviors when it comes to relationships.

A child raised by attentive caregivers will develop a healthy sense of interdependence with others. Attachment with primary caregivers very much influences the way we view ourselves and our worth. If my primary caregivers, those people who are biologically programmed to love me, send unspoken messages that I lack value and worth, why would I think that I am worthy of love? The answer, of course, is that our primary caregivers do not determine our worth.

Yet, we rarely challenge our internal messages. We accept them as true, while assuming there must be some inherent authority to our internal knowledge. However, when our information about ourselves is built on faulty beliefs and experiences, it is as unreliable as the caregivers on whom we were initially forced to rely.

It is important that you realize that our worth as individuals is inherent simply because we exist. None of us are here by mistake. We each have a unique set of gifts, talents, and qualities bestowed upon us. It is our responsibility to learn what they are and use them to the best of our ability. Exploring our belief system is a crucial step to emotional well-being. A healthy belief system allows us to identify our purpose and to live it. *Beliefs provide the meaning that guide our purpose.*

Many people in our society have suffered abuse in childhood, whether it is sexual, physical, verbal, emotional, spiritual, or a function of neglect. Emotional neglect is particularly insidious because it is difficult to identify and articulate yet it is incredibly damaging. It is the absence of "something" in childhood that causes pain, and because children have a very small frame of reference, it is impossible to identify until much later in life. Young children do not say to their parents, "You are not meeting my emotional needs and you are violating my boundaries." Children do not have the understanding to articulate what they are experiencing, so they act out instead. Behind unwanted behaviors in children is usually deeply rooted emotional pain. Often, children who demonstrate the worst behaviors are the ones who need the most understanding, love, and healing.

Emotional neglect and abuse can be difficult to identify with specificity. What is damaging to one child may not register for another child. A good rule of thumb is – if you experienced it as hurtful, it was impactful and harmful to you in some way. That impact is a sufficient reason to begin the process of healing childhood wounds.

When abuse is perpetrated against a child, both psychological changes and physiological changes occur. The message that is sent to a child who is being sexually abused is, "My need for sexual gratification is more important than your well-being, and, therefore, your existence." This lack of importance, in comparison to others sends the message that, "You are worthless. You have no value." Remember, children have simplistic concepts of the world that equate to: if it's happening to me and it's bad – it's my fault.

These beliefs that are created as the abuse occurs create enduring personal philosophies that are difficult to modify. When abuse occurs, a core belief has been instilled in a very permanent way. These beliefs are reinforced with recurring abuse. In turn, reinforcement further solidifies the belief. The resulting negative internal dialog further reinforces this belief system and it becomes entrenched - so much so, that it becomes a part of who we are.

As the child goes forward in life, the brain is wired to accept information that confirms what we believe to be true and reject information that does not fit with what we believe. Think about how hard it is to change someone else's mind! It is equally as difficult to change our own beliefs when they become entrenched as a function of our negative experiences.

For a child who has experienced abuse, events such as failing a quiz, forgetting something, rejection by a romantic interest, not making a school sports team all equate to confirmations of unworthiness, unlovability, and inadequacy. Compliments, successes, and romantic interests all become anomalies or may be interpreted as nefariously motived because of our negative experiences with others.

Perhaps you can begin to see the lifelong, deep psychological damage abuse renders on the survivor. This phenomenon is why people can't just "get over it" simply because "it was a long time ago." These pronouncements often come from friends or loved ones who are attempting to motivate the person to move on. They often come from a place of frustration when loved ones feel helpless to render aid or assistance. Our damaged and distorted beliefs are the nagging residue of unresolved trauma and they fuel unhealthy emotions and behaviors. In that way, we perpetuate the pain of the abuse by continuing to visit it upon ourselves. In fact, we often generate the isolation that confirms our unworthiness.

People mistakenly believe that two events need to occur in order to heal: acknowledgment of harm by the perpetrator and subsequent forgiveness. Sometimes perpetrators are not available or they have passed away. Perpetrators rarely admit their actions, rarely show remorse, and are rarely capable of the insight necessary to fully comprehend the deleterious and lasting impact of their actions. Encounters and letters to perpetrators can actually have the opposite effect and serve to further victimize and traumatize the survivor because of the perpetrator's lack of acknowledgment or remorse. In an effort to seek healing and in the absence of acknowledgment by the perpetrator, people often seek understanding from others under the guise of "I need people to know my truth."

However, contrary to popular maxims, forgiveness is not the impetus for healing. What is really needed for healing is the processing of the trauma (beyond the scope of this book) and challenging and replacing the damaged belief system with a healthy, appropriate one. Validation from others only goes so far. It may help you feel better in the moment, but it is not a long-term solution to your pain.

Not surprisingly, forgiveness frequently comes after self-healing. It is much easier to discover a desire for forgiveness once healing has begun and painful, raw, intense emotions begin to subside. We will explore forgiveness further on Day 30. For now, it is important to know that forgiveness contributes to our happiness. However, this only occurs only after much other work has been done. Let's do that work and return to the topic when we are better able to forgive (for our own sake). For now, just remember, a desire to forgive will harken you once sufficient healing has occurred.

Damage to the functioning of the brain and the nervous system also occurs during childhood. During traumatic events, soft tissue damage can occur in the hippocampus, which wires the brain for fear. When a brain experiences a severe threat or a potentially life threatening event, the brain switches to a state of high alert. The brain becomes wired for fear, which is the essence of post-traumatic stress disorder and often presents as anxiety. Screening for trauma is an important task for mental health professionals when assessing a client. This approach is called "trauma-informed" and today many healthcare professionals are approaching patients and clients from a trauma-informed perspective.

Role of Shame and Blame

An important concept to understand about childhood abuse, especially sexual abuse, is the transfer of shame and blame to the survivor during the course of the abuse. Let's explore these mechanisms, why they are a common denominator in abuse survivors, and why they linger into adulthood.

Remember that during abuse, situations are confusing and chaotic, especially when there is severe physical abuse, neglect, and/or sexual abuse. Our brains are naturally wired to make sense of what we are experiencing. In the absence of an explanation that makes sense to our brains, our brains will fill in the gaps of information. Abuse often begins during developmental periods of egocentrism in children when children are formatively incapable of differentiating themselves from others and when they are only capable of associating events with themselves. The child brain makes sense of something bad happening with an explanation that they are bad. The child brain says to itself, "I'm bad, which is why something bad is happening to me."

The intensity of the experience hard-wires the belief into the brain and it becomes a very strong pathway to which current experiences revert, and shame is born. Remember from earlier sessions, shame is the "I am" experience. Going forward, each new experience is compared to this powerful belief system. When a powerful negative belief system is present, a resulting emotion is shame and it is felt with the overwhelming intensity of the original experience.

Another mechanism of brain function which fuels damaged belief systems is the meaning-making orientation of our brains. We are biologically driven to seek understanding from our experiences. Our brains are wired to process information when it is complete. Traumatic experiences are chaotic and the information available to victims/survivors is incomplete and illogical. "What is happening?" and "What caused this event?" are two questions the brain needs to know to understand the event and process it from short-term to long-term memory. In the absence of information, our brains will look for information in the environment in order to make sense of the event. To fill the information gap, the child brain will utilize its only point of reference, itself, and ask itself what it possibly could have done.

For example, if a child experiences a parent hitting them, screaming in their face, and verbally abusing them over a messy room, the child will naturally make the assumption that failing to complete a task (cleaning the room sufficiently and in a timely manner) was the cause of the abuse when, in fact, the parent is the source of the abuse. Think about a parent who does not pay attention when a child speaks and shows no interest in their accomplishments but notes the accomplishments of other children. The child's interpretation may be that they need to be perfect in order to be loved and accepted, again, not recognizing the parent's responsibility and failure.

The brain's orientation of requiring an explanation for events is the source of self-blame. These self-recriminations evolve from "I did" which fuels blame and guilt, to "I am" which fuels shame. It often takes experiences well into adulthood to challenge these beliefs. Since these beliefs were formed in relationships, they surface in relationships. Intimate relationships are fertile ground for maladaptive beliefs to surface in problematic ways. We will explore relationships further on Day 27.

Remember, truly healing from abuse and traumatic events is beyond the scope of one book. A skilled and talented therapist can help and *you are worthy of help and healing*.

We will begin the healing journey of childhood abuse by exploring the damaged belief system. Use the childhood abuse beliefs worksheet to begin to identify what statements are part of your belief system. Review the 'Negative' column and put a check mark next the statements that apply to you. In the next column, begin to identify replacement statements that can become part of your new belief system. There is room at the bottom for your own additions.

A final note about abuse: being honest with yourself that people you love were abusive is not a betrayal. This process is not about blame – it is about healing and recovery and you are worth it!

CHILDHOOD ABUSE BELIEFS WORKSHEET

NEGATIVE	POSITIVE
I am inherently unlovable	I have inherent value and worth
I am damaged	I am lovable
I am broken	I am whole and okay
I am not normal	I am okay even if I feel negative emotions
I am not likable	My emotions are not who I am
There is something wrong with me	I love myself, flaws and all
I am different	My flaws and imperfections make me interesting
I don't matter	My flaws just mean I have room to grow
I am not important	I will not fall to pieces if someone criticizes me
I have no value and worth	Whoever I share my life with is lucky
I need to get them first	I have many gifts, talents, and qualities
I have to be perfect to be loved	My childhood abuse does not define me
I am weird	My childhood abuse is not who I am
I can't make mistakes	My childhood abuse is something that happened to me
I am ugly	I am healing
I am a failure	Mistakes are learning tools
I am a loser	I am a work in progress
I am stupid	I can learn new skills and tasks
I am not good at anything	I can change
I should get over it	I am free
I should be happy	I am in control of my destiny
I have no control	I am not defined by my accomplishments
I will never be able to change	I have purpose
I am not good enough	I am special
I will never accomplish anything	I am unique
I will never be successful	I can feel joy
I will never be happy	I can have a great life
I am invisible	I deserve a great life
I am nothing special	I deserve to be loved
People will always hurt me	I am allowed to set healthy boundaries with others
People will always leave me	I am capable
People will abandon me	I am intelligent
People are not trustworthy	I can control my thoughts, beliefs, and emotions
No one will ever truly love me	I can keep going
Other people are better than I am	I am an amazing person
Nothing ever works out for me	I can make a difference
Other people define me	I don't need to earn love from people
I am hopeless	I am awesome

HOMEWORK DAY 5

1) Utilizing the Childhood Abuse Beliefs worksheet, identify negative beliefs, identify positive beliefs that you say to yourself, and identify positive beliefs that you want to incorporate into your personal belief system.

2) Complete an ABC worksheet on any situation.

3) Make a commitment to complete Day 6.

KEEP IT GOING!!!

DAY 6 CHALLENGING BELIEFS

Today's Objectives: 1) Begin the process of identifying and challenging damaging, negative beliefs 2) Begin to establish a new, healthy, realistic belief system

Today's lesson is an expansion of Day 1, ABC worksheets. In the ABC worksheet process, you will recall the reframing process whereby we identified a thought distortion and reframed it into a more helpful thought process. In today's lesson, we will expand the reframing process in order to more deeply challenge the negative thought.

As discussed in previous lessons, many of our negative beliefs are deeply ingrained and difficult to change. These beliefs were formatively created and we have reinforced them by repeating them as truths to ourselves, time and time again over years and sometimes decades. For this reason, we hold them as absolute truths when they are, in fact, falsehoods that directionally misguide us and ultimately misalign us with others.

These deeply held beliefs are generated and confirmed by our primary caregivers and reinforced by our experiences. Our brains are designed to accept confirming information and reject conflicting information. Because of this dynamic, changing unhealthy beliefs is a difficult task. New thoughts and beliefs feel strange, uncertain, untrue, and unreliable at first. Repeated practice and continual exposure to the new belief system is necessary to generate meaningful change.

In today's lesson, we will make use of the Challenging My Beliefs worksheet to assist with the process of creating a healthy belief system.

In the first column of the worksheet, "What I Tell Myself," identify a negative thought or belief -- something you say to yourself about yourself. You can use an unhelpful thought identified in one of your ABC worksheets, use one you identified in yesterday's lesson, or you can use a new one.

In the second column, "Proof That This Is True," see if you can identify any factual evidence to support your belief. What is the factual evidence that this belief is true?

For example, if my belief is "I am inherently unlovable," what is the factual evidence that this belief is true? Remember, we are looking for FACTUAL evidence. Just because someone does not love me, that fact does not make me unlovable. Did you love everyone you had a relationship with? Do you love everyone you meet?

Consider a situation where someone was heartbroken then moved on to a new, successful relationship. After the breakup, was that person unlovable? No! They may have been unloved by a particular person, but that does not make the person unlovable.

It's time to see yourself the same way. If, for some reason, you are currently unloved or unloved by someone in particular, it does not make you unlovable.

In the middle column, "Where Did This Belief Come From," begin to explore the origin of your negative belief. See if you can identify events in your past that sent an underlying negative message, such as bullying. Painful childhood experiences are a great place to begin your search for origins of negative beliefs. Also, consider influential people in your life, including parents, siblings, teachers, friends, and other family members. The purpose of this column is not to place blame or to criticize, but rather to begin to make connections, facilitate understanding, and to promote healing.

Messages received early in our lives have a very powerful influence on our constructed sense of self because we have little or no ability to question them. As discussed in yesterday's lesson, Childhood Abuse, we accept them as true without any filtering or evaluative processes. We then incorporate and weave them into the fabric of our being. Now is your opportunity to explore the origins of your constructed sense of self, possibly for the first time.

Emotional responses, including anger, are an expected part of this exercise and represent an important part of the process. If needed, take a moment and use the Unhelpful Emotions word list to identify your feelings. Keep in mind that feeling these unpleasant emotions is probably a part of your healing journey!

The fourth column, "Proof That This Is Not True," is the opposite of the second column, "Proof That This Is True." Identify factual evidence that is contrary to your belief in column 1. Look in your life for specific examples that are contrary to the identified belief.

It may seem incorrect to use factual evidence in this column that is counter to evidence from column 2. It is possible for evidence to both support and refute a belief.

For example, it is possible to challenge a belief that I am unlovable by looking for examples of being loved while, simultaneously, not allowing examples of people who do not love me to support that same belief.

As we incorporate these concepts into our daily lives, we begin to take things less personally. When we start the process of not taking things personally, it allows room for us to create our own, healthy constructed sense of self that is positive yet realistic.

You have the ability to decide who you are, what you stand for, and create an integrated, whole sense of self. We will continue to explore our identity on Day 26.

In the last column of the worksheet, "New Belief," see if you can identify a new, healthy statement. Feel free to use statements from yesterday's lesson. See if you can state a belief positively about yourself – don't just add 'not,' such as "I'm not a loser."

Remember, these new beliefs feel awkward and strange at first. However, using this process of challenging old beliefs will usher in new ones because you will witness first-hand how illogical some of your core beliefs actually are. This exercise begins the process of accepting and endorsing a new belief system that is more attuned to your experiences as a whole.

CHALLENGING MY BELIEFS

WHAT I TELL MYSELF	PROOF THAT THIS IS TRUE	WHERE DID THIS BELIEF COME FROM?	PROOF THAT THIS BELIEF IS NOT TRUE	NEW BELIEF
Example: *I am unlovable.*	*My husband left me.* *My boyfriend broke up with me.*	*My mother treated me like I was unlovable.* *I could never do anything right as a kid.*	*My dad loves me. My kids love me. I have dated people who loved me.*	*I am lovable even if not everyone loves me. If someone doesn't love me, it is their opinion, not a fact that I am not worthy of love.*

HOMEWORK DAY 6

1) Complete the Challenging My Beliefs worksheet. Begin to incorporate new beliefs in your thinking patterns.

2) Complete an ABC worksheet on any situation.

3) Make a commitment to complete Day 7.

YOU GOT THIS!!!

DAY 7 DAILY GRATITUDE

Today's Objective: Learn the process of changing your world view to begin to see the world through a lens of gratitude and generate positivity and true happiness.

The concept of having "an attitude of gratitude" has been popularized, in part, because there is some science behind it. Thoughts of gratitude actually activate the brain's reward center and trigger a host of chemicals, while also boosting bonds with other people. Gratitude can ease depression and anxiety symptoms and improve sleep, mainly due to the replacement of negative thoughts and the reduction of stress hormones they generate.

Gratitude activates the hypothalamus, which is responsible for regulating such functions as hunger, sleep, body temperature, and metabolism. Feeling grateful or doing something altruistic activates the limbic system of the brain and causes various bodily functions to operate more efficiently. Gratitude helps the brain become more resilient, or bounce back from stressful situations, which reduces stress overall.

And finally, the mechanisms of gratitude rely on the prefrontal cortex, which is one of the areas in the brain responsible for memory formation. Thoughts of gratitude are retained as positive information in this part of the brain, which serves to negate negative thought processes. In this way, the brain is literally retrained to be positive, resulting in higher levels of happiness.

Those who practice gratitude are more likely to achieve goals, to be more generous, be less self-centered, be more respectful, and to be less judgmental.

You may, if you like, keep a written gratitude journal. Alternatively, you may wish to choose someone you are close to like a spouse, partner, friend, parent, sibling, or child and send a daily selfie along with your daily gratitude. This approach helps with grounding, builds relationships, and promotes accountability. A few small suggestions for your gratitude expressions:

1) State one thing you are grateful for. Try to go beyond material possessions.

2) State why you are grateful. This part is the most important aspect of the exercise because it is where the thought and feeling actually occur and get encoded in the brain.

3) Do not repeat anything you have identified. Find something new every day to be grateful for.

You will notice that the exercise is fairly easy for the first week or two, then you really have to search for things in your life to be grateful for. You will also notice that you begin to take neutral or negative encounters and develop the ability to see the positive, gratitude-based side of the overall experience.

Here is an example:

While at a cocktail party at a friend's house, someone hit my car and totaled it. There are so many aspects of this situation to be grateful for. 1) I knew who did it and he gave me his insurance information and apologized. I'm grateful it wasn't a hit and run, which would have caused me to make a claim on my insurance. 2) I'm grateful he wasn't hurt. I'm grateful no one was standing nearby and got hurt. I'm grateful I wasn't in the car. I'm grateful my family wasn't in the car. Cars can be replaced. People can't! 3) I'm grateful the car was totaled and not fixed. The car would have lost value and it would have been more difficult to resell a car that had had substantial damage to it. 4) I'm grateful I received a rental car and the process was smooth and easy. 5) I'm grateful for the supportive response from my friends. Everyone at the party expressed concern and many offered to take me home after the party. 6) I'm grateful I have a great party story for years to come!

That evening, many people commented on my lack of reaction during the event and commented that they would not have remained so calm. It was just a car. My mind instantly went to a place of gratitude about the various aspects of the situation listed above. Gratitude works!

Here are some ways to practice gratitude, use the exercise outlined above, or use the gratitude worksheet.

Ways to Practice Gratitude:

Give thanks and appreciation to yourself for something.

Give thanks for your meal.

Build a gratitude board.

Read books on cultivating gratitude.

Place a gratitude evocative word card or note in sight, such as a bathroom mirror.

Use a special object as a seed for gratitude meditation.

Find value, meaning, and purpose from suffering.

Thank your body with a massage or a bath ritual.

Send notes and cards of appreciation and thanks to others.

Move and dance with gratitude.

Give thanks with a random act of kindness.

Develop a nightly gratitude ritual.

Have family members identify daily gratitude before dinner.

Send a prayer of thanks to people in your life.

Let someone know when they inspire you.

Make a gratitude jar with daily notes.

Journal your gratitude.

Draw a picture that is an expression of gratitude.

Keep in mind that gratitude reduces negativity. If you have a family member, pet, or co-worker, who has an annoying habit – you may tend to focus on it. If you find things to be grateful for about the object of your frustration, you will feel less frustrated.

DATE	DAILY GRATITUDE	WHY

HOMEWORK DAY 7

QUOTE OF THE DAY:

IF WE DON'T FEEL GRATEFUL WITH WHAT WE ALREADY HAVE, WHAT MAKES US THINK WE WILL BE HAPPY WITH MORE? – SUKH SANDHU

1) Begin daily gratitude exercise.

2) Complete an ABC worksheet on any situation.

3) Make a commitment to complete Day 8.

WEEK ONE DOWN! ONTO THE NEXT WEEK!!!

DAY 8 PATTERNS OF THINKING

Today's Objective: 1) Learn patterns of thinking that contribute to negative and distorted emotional and behavioral responses 2) Use patterns of thinking categories to further challenge thought distortions identified in previous lessons

In today's lesson, we will continue to delve into challenging the way we think by looking at patterns of thinking in conjunction with the cognitive process outlined in the ABC worksheet. When we recognize our patterns of thinking, this awareness will enable us to change stubborn thought processes that undermine our happiness and well-being. In essence, we are thinking about thinking.

We will review some common thought patterns and distortions, then use a worksheet to ascertain where our negative thinking patterns exist, and then identify necessary changes that need to be made.

TYPES OF THINKING PATTERNS

Assuming

The first pattern of thinking is assuming, which can involve mindreading or fortune telling. With assuming, the worst possible scenario is imagined, often without valid evidence or facts. For many people, especially those with difficult childhoods or trauma experiences, assuming patterns develop as a result of the survival mechanisms in the brain. If I can mentally play out various scenarios and prepare for the worst-case scenario, I will increase my chances of being prepared, and thus, improve my chances of survival. With mindreading, one assumes they know what someone else is thinking. Alternatively, with fortune telling, one assumes they can predict future events. In both instances, negative assumptions are made.

Examples: 1) My boyfriend decides to go out with his friends. I assume he is planning to cheat on me or preparing to leave me (Mindreading). 2) I made a huge mistake at work. I forgot to put in a special materials order for our biggest customer. I will be fired (Fortune Telling).

Solution: Look for all possible explanations and consider the most likely one. Do not dwell on the worst-case scenario.

Shoulds/Musts/Oughts

If *shoulds* or *musts* creep into our vocabulary, we are engaging in negative comparisons. These thought patterns keep us in a "lesser than" position, in that they make us feel inferior and they cause us to ignore our progress and achievements. Because the use of *should* and *must* involves negative comparison, this type of thinking induces guilt and/or shame. Similarly, *ought* thought patterns involve the same negative comparisons of others, which induces feelings of frustration, anger, and resentment toward them. By using *should* or *must* in our thought processes, we effectively demotivate ourselves. When using *ought* in our thought process, we are priming ourselves for resentment.

Examples: 1) I should have worked out longer than I did today. 2) I should be married and have kids by now. 3) He ought to appreciate me more for all the help I gave him.

Solution: Replace 'should' or 'must' with 'could' or 'would.' Replace 'ought' with "I would prefer if he or she would/could..."

Fairy Tale Fantasy

Similar to *shoulds/musts/oughts*, the fairy tale fantasy involves the expectation that life *should be fair*. When a situation unfolds that is not fair, individuals who expect fairness respond with distress and their thoughts center on the unfairness or injustice of the situation. Alternatively, individuals who do not approach life with the expectation of fairness, respond to the same situation by exploring solutions. In reality, life is not fair – bad things happen to good people. Difficulties, even tragedies, happen randomly, as a consequence of neglect, unreasonableness, malevolence of others, or as a function of our own mistakes or shortcomings. A lack of acceptance of our situation or our status in life invites disappointment or distress. Moreover, it is the expectation that leads to distress and disappointment more than the situation itself.

Examples: 1) It's not fair that he got the promotion because of his family's connections. 2) I am much more deserving of a good man than she is. It's just not fair.

Solution: Focus on acceptance of yourself, others, and situations. Place events in life into one of two categories – things I can control and things I cannot control. By accepting aspects of life that you cannot control, you alleviate distress and modulate your disappointment. Therefore, it is best to monitor and curb unrealistic expectations.

Black and White

This thinking pattern involves seeing ourselves, others, or situations dichotomously – only two possible choices exist. Something is either good or bad, right or wrong, all or nothing. This view permits no room for other explanations and often eliminates the ability to consider situational context. This thinking pattern is common in trauma survivors. When information is processed quickly and dichotomously, it affords quick reactions that promote survival in extreme situations. Time spent on the nuances or in shades of grey represent a threat to survival, in the moment. For the trauma brain, time is of the essence in order to ensure survival. It is more expedient to consider two explanations than ten possibilities. People with trauma histories tend to get stuck in this reactive stance, and they often remain unaware of the shift in their thinking patterns.

Examples: 1) A friend lets you down by forgetting a lunch date and you conclude they are untrustworthy. 2) A prospective romantic interest reveals she cheated on a previous boyfriend and she is unilaterally dismissed as a serial cheater who cannot be faithful.

Solution: Recognize all-or-nothing thought processes, begin using words such as 'some' or 'sometimes.' Begin to consider more than two options as solutions or possible scenarios. Begin to ponder alternate explanations that allow room for context.

Overgeneralizing

This thought pattern involves seeing one negative event as a future guarantee of the same experience. One negative engagement is seen as an inevitable and inescapable future. Overgeneralizing statements often include words like "never", "always", "all", and "every". Absolutes rarely occur in the real world. When absolute statements creep into your vocabulary, you are likely overgeneralizing.

Examples: 1) Thoughts such as 'things never go my way.' 2) "One bad blind date means all blind dates are bad."

Solution: Recognize that unrelated events, such as different blind dates or different people, do not all share a common pattern. However, patterns do exist in individuals, such as a friend who always runs late. These patterns do not need to be ignored, but make sure that 'all' and 'always' assumptions are challenged. In the real world, it rarely (if ever) happens that way.

Labeling

This pattern involves describing ourselves, others, and situations with negative words. Humans are complex beings and a one-word descriptor does not represent the entirety of an individual. Often, the word used to describe a person, more aptly applies to their behavior in a given situation. Keep in mind, identification and categorization are ways our mind helps us survive. They have an evolutionary basis because we cannot relive every encounter as if it is new without gaining something from our previous experiences. On the other hand, we should be mindful of global labels that we use to define ourselves or others on the basis of a single quality or our/others behavior/performance at one moment in time.

Examples: 1) I am such a loser. 2) He is stupid.

Solution: Focus on behaviors instead of people or situations, such as 'that was a silly thing to do.'

Dwelling on the Negative

This thought pattern is also the result of the survival mechanisms in our brain. Negative information is more relevant for survival than positive information. This explanation offers insight into why human beings remember insults and dismiss compliments as superfluous. Furthermore, for those with difficult childhoods or trauma survivors, our brains are primed to be keen on negative situational aspects. After all, focusing on negative information or threatening aspects of a situation to assess for safety is critical to survival. On the other hand, remaining focused on the negative, when the actual threat has passed, interferes with our ability to be happy and wholeheartedly engage the world. Trauma survivors often unwittingly slip into this pattern of thinking without recognizing the shift. Doing an honest accounting of your thought processes is the first step to favorably altering the way you experience the world.

Examples: 1) Overcooking the vegetables and viewing the entire meal as an epic failure. 2) Focusing on the glitches or problems when recounting a vacation.

Solution: Focus on all aspects of people or situations. Try balancing an equal number of positive and negative thoughts or comments. Find something to be positive about, even in a negative situation. If nothing else, events in life occur in degrees and most situations could actually have been worse. (Remember your daily gratitude!)

Rejecting the Positive

Dismissing or negating positive information is the counterpart to the previous pattern and these patterns often occur in conjunction. Rejecting compliments is often derived from low self-esteem and, as a result, accomplishments are not enjoyed. When we dismiss positive experiences, we maintain negative beliefs that are actually contradicted by our daily experiences. In the long run, we can actually lose touch with reality when we hyper focus on the negative and discount the positive.

Examples: 1) 'Oh, this old thing! I've had it for ages and I got it on sale. I feel fat in it.' 2) 'I'm sure he doesn't think I'm pretty. He probably has other motives.'

Solution: Think of a compliment as a gift and say 'thank you.' Allow yourself to savor and enjoy your achievements and accomplishments.

Unfavorable Comparisons

In this thought distortion, we compare ourselves to someone or something else in a singular category or in a particular way whereby the self is comparatively inferior. Our own qualities, traits, or strengths are minimized and our mistakes or faults are magnified; meanwhile, the strengths of others are enhanced and their mistakes are minimized. When comparing ourselves to someone or something else, the quality or situation under inspection is observed singularly, and out of context, and we assess ourselves as inferior or inadequate by comparison. In reality, examining only one aspect of someone, something, or a situation is out of context and this lack of perspective leads to faulty conclusions.

Examples: 1) They seem so happy together as a couple (ignoring that their finances are a mess). 2) She is always dressed so nicely and I always look frumpy.

Solution: Stand on your own, do not compare yourself to others. Living life to the fullest is about being the best you that you can be and that does not arise from constant comparisons to others. If you must compare yourself, remember that everyone has their faults or shortcomings. Recognize where you are minimizing yourself and learn to celebrate the good and unique qualities/characteristics of you.

Catastrophizing

This pattern is another common adaptation by those with difficult childhoods or trauma experiences. We anticipate disaster and we contemplate the worst possible outcome. It is effectively a preemptive strike, by preparing for the worst possibility, we hope to avoid the surprise, victimization, and disappointment of our past. These anticipated situations are viewed as intolerable and we believe we are/will be unable to cope or manage the situation, our emotions, or our behaviors. We view the situation as permanent, rather than temporary, and we are unable to formulate an action plan in order to manage it. In many ways, this involves being stuck in the victimization of our past, and it is another adaptation in thought that unknowingly creeps into the emotional repertoire of trauma survivors.

Examples: 1) My car accident is the worst thing that could ever happen. 2) Because of my divorce, my life is over.

Solution: Realistically assess the odds of an event occurring, if it hasn't happened yet. If it does happen, consider what range of possibilities exists? How can you minimize its impact? What plan of action can you create to avoid being overwhelmed in the moment? Put the event in perspective - will this situation matter a week, a month, or a year from now?

Personalizing

This pattern involves seeing ourselves as more involved in a situation than may actually be true. It encompasses believing that what others say or do is somehow a direct, personal reaction to you. In this pattern, our ego, or constructed sense of self, is seen as being at the center of situations. When we are pivotal to the issue or event, it becomes a challenge to our self-worth. Correlations are not distinguished from causations and outside influences are not considered. Personalization can also involve self-blame. Self-blame arises from holding oneself accountable or responsible for events outside of your control.

Examples: 1) My brother slighted me by completely ignoring my advice. 2) The cashier was deliberately rude to me. How dare she treat me that way! 3). It's my fault my husband cheats on me. If I were a better partner, that would not happen.

Solution: Recognize that nothing in this world is personal. Everyone acts from their own needs all the time. Look for alternate explanations to assist in recognizing the difference between taking something personally and experiencing a situation that personally impacts you. Someone hitting my car is not personal but it will affect me personally. My partner cheating on me is not my fault but it will personally impact me.

Blaming

This pattern is the opposite of personalizing and involves placing responsibility on someone or something outside the self. In this pattern, the ego is usually so fragile, one cannot take responsibility and is unable to separate the self from the behavior. When presented with the prospect of owning the mistake, the entire self is seen as bad rather than acknowledging the choice or behavior as bad and understanding that one act does not define anyone.

Examples: 1) She makes me angry! 2) My boss doesn't like me so I will never get ahead.

Solution: Begin to take ownership of behaviors while keeping your self-worth intact. Ironically, the more responsibility you take for behaviors, the more in control and powerful you will feel. We give our personal power away when we decide that others determine our fate.

Making Feelings Facts

In this thinking pattern, feelings are accepted as unrefuted proof of a thought or a situation. Now that you are becoming an ABC worksheet aficionado, you know that feelings arise from thoughts - not the reverse. Feelings are not facts.

Examples: 1) I feel like a loser so I *am* a loser. 2) Flying must be dangerous and unsafe because I feel anxious getting on a plane.

Solution: Recognize that thoughts precede feelings. Thought distortions cause negative emotional responses. Look for factual evidence in a situation rather than accepting feelings as factual proof. Feelings are a signal that you need to explore how you are thinking.

In today's worksheet, the thinking patterns are listed in the left-hand column. You may not employ every type of distorted thinking. You may be prone to one thinking error in a specific area of your life, such as a family situation. In the middle column, identify specific examples of the pattern in your life. In the right-hand column, see if you can identify a healthier alternative to the thought pattern. If you have difficulty with an alternative thought, look back at the suggestions on how to overcome specific thinking errors.

PATTERNS OF THINKING WORKSHEET

Type of Thought	Example	Replacement
Assuming		
Shoulds/Musts/Oughts		
Fairy-Tale Fantasy		
Black and White		
Overgeneralizing		
Labeling		
Dwelling on the Negative		
Rejecting the Positive		
Unfavorable Comparisons		
Catastrophizing		
Personalizing		
Blaming		
Making Feelings Facts		

HOMEWORK DAY 8

1) Complete Patterns of Thinking worksheet.

2) Identify daily gratitude.

3) Complete an ABC worksheet on any situation.

4) Make a commitment to complete Day 9.

YOU CAN DO IT!!!

DAY 9 COMMUNICATION

Today's Objective: 1) Learn a simple framework for expressing ourselves in a healthy, effective manner 2) Learn the difference between passive, aggressive, passive-aggressive, and assertive communication 3) Assess your assertiveness 4) Begin to improve your assertiveness 5) Begin to implement healthy forms of communication

Most of us have heard the axiom, 'It's not what you say, but how you say it.' In today's lesson, we will be working on the latter half of that statement. Improving how we communicate with others promotes understanding in human interactions, thereby improving relationships. When we improve our interactions, we build relationship skills and solidify relationships, which is crucial to our overall well-being.

Many aspects of who we are, including patterns of relating to others, are modeled for us by our family of origin and rooted in early childhood experiences. We learn to communicate with others by having our primary caregivers communicate with us, and by watching them communicate with others.

When unhealthy communication patterns are modeled for us (as were modeled for them, and so on), we, in turn, carry on the generational legacy of unhealthy and ineffective communication patterns. These patterns are counterproductive and sometimes even toxic.

Today's lesson is an opportunity to modify undesirable legacies and begin communicating more effectively and productively.

We will begin by learning a basic framework for communicating. As we proceed, remember - a behavior is something someone does or doesn't do, says or doesn't say.

```
When you _____
              (behavior)
I feel/I felt _____
              (feeling)

Optional:

Because _____

Optional:

I want you to _____
```

In this template, the first two lines are key. Rather than attacking a person or their character, we will begin to focus on behaviors and how they make us feel. If there is a reason that needs to be explained, add a 'because' statement. In order to improve understanding between individuals, add an 'I want you to' or 'I would prefer' or 'it would be helpful' statement.

Here are some examples to consider:

Instead of: Quit interrupting me. You never shut up.

Try: When you interrupt me, I feel frustrated and marginalized because it makes me feel like you don't respect what I have to say. I want you to listen until I am finished speaking.

Instead of: You're ignoring me.

Try: When you are looking at your cell phone when I try to talk to you, I feel ignored and unimportant because your phone seems more important than I am. I would prefer if you would put your phone down and look at me when I talk to you.

Instead of: Do you think you could be on time for once?

Try: I get frustrated when you are late because my time is important. I would prefer if you would shoot me a quick text to let me know.

Other Behaviors That Improve Communication

Address chronic, problematic behaviors instead of ignoring them.

Refrain from addressing issues while still angry or heated.

Refrain from using "You need to…"

Refrain from name-calling or using "You are…." (i.e. lazy, selfish, dumb).

Refrain from talking over others.

Avoid distracting comments.

Acknowledge the feelings, comments, opinions of others.

Ask open-ended questions, such as, "Tell me about…" or "How do you feel about…"

Be specific, avoid generalizations.

Refrain from sarcasm.

THE FOUR COMMUNICATION STYLES

Passive

Characteristics: Passive communicators avoid expressing their own opinion, identifying their own needs, or defending their own rights. It is the absence of communication or excessive submission in an effort to avoid being considered disagreeable. To circumvent negative impressions of them, these communicators avoid communicating their feelings or concerns and excessively submit in an effort to appear agreeable. Generally, this style arises from a lack of confidence that is borne from difficult childhoods. Passive communicators often feel lonely and isolated because they keep their thoughts, feelings, and experiences to themselves.

Beliefs: I'm not as important as others.
No one cares what I think.
No one cares about my feelings.
What I say is unimportant.
If I speak up, people will be mad and leave/reject me.
I'm not allowed to have rights.

Behaviors: Apologizing, minimizing
Failure to assert themselves
Failure to express themselves
Limited eye contact, slumped posture
Soft spoken, quiet

Results: Allows others to take advantage
Anxiety and depression
Feelings of powerlessness, hopelessness
Development of resentment
Avoidance, excuses
Use of defense mechanisms

Examples: "That's ok."
"I don't mind."
"Sure."
"No problem."
"Whatever you need."
"I'm happy with what everyone else wants."

Aggressive

Characteristics: Aggressive communicators express themselves in a way that violates the rights of others. Ironically, aggressive communicators also often develop from difficult childhoods. Temperaments (discussed on Day 19) often play a role in communication style, as well as other factors, such as modeling. Often, underneath an aggressive communication style is deep pain, hurt, and fear.

Beliefs: I demand to be heard.
Other people's feelings and thoughts don't matter.
I have a right to violate your rights.
Your rights don't matter.
I'm superior to you.
You are inferior to me.
It's your fault.
I'm not at fault.

Behaviors: Easily frustrated, outwardly agitated
Loud, threatening, demanding tone
Profanity, name calling
Poor listening
Frequently interrupts
Uses criticism, humiliation, and domination
Blames others, makes excuses
Uses 'you' statements, as well as 'always' and 'never'
Intense eye contact, physical intimidation

Results: Anxiety and depression
Becomes alienated from others
Feelings of powerfulness intermingled with feelings of hopelessness
Use of defense mechanisms
High blood pressure, physical manifestations of disease

Examples: "I don't care what you want."
"Shut up."
"You are an idiot and don't know what you're talking about."
"You never listen to me."
"You better do what I say."
"If you don't do what I want, you will regret it."

Passive-Aggressive

Characteristics: This style involves indirect aggression via a seemingly passive style of communication. The aggressive aspect of this style can include the absence of communication (shutting down), subtle or indirect communication, or surreptitious communication. As with the first two styles, individuals who experience difficult childhoods, and those with families of origin who modeled this style, will utilize passive-aggressive forms of communication.

Beliefs: I'm weak so I need to communicate in other ways (sabotage, frustrate, insinuate).
I'm going to pretend to be agreeable but I'm not.
I can't win directly but I will indirectly.
I'm powerless now but I will regain my power in other ways.
This behavior is the only way I can get my point across.

Behaviors: Excessive sarcasm
Condescending tone
Use of denial
Failure to speak (stonewalling)
Verbalize agreement then reverse positions
Use of sabotage
Feign ignorance or incompetence
Muttering

Results: Anxiety and depression
Becomes alienated from others
Avoidance, blaming, excuses
Development of resentment
Distrustful

Examples: "Fine."
"Whatever."
"I was just kidding."
"I'm not sure why you are so angry."
"You look good for someone your age."

Assertive

Characteristics: Assertive communicators respectfully consider the needs, feelings, thoughts, and opinions of all individuals as mutually important. This style is characterized by confidence, a willingness to compromise, active listening, and effective communication. Those with good self-esteem express themselves assertively.

Beliefs: I am important, but no more or less important than others.
I can't control others but I can control myself.
We are all entitled to express ourselves in a respectful manner.
The rights, values, opinions, feelings, and needs of others are just as important as mine.
I have a right to express myself.
I'm responsible for my own happiness.

Behaviors: Uses healthy communication skills
Uses calm, clear voice
Clearly states wants, needs, feelings, thoughts, beliefs
Willing to compromise
Exudes confidence
Good eye contact, open body posture
Listens without interrupting
Communicates respect for others

Results: Feels connected to others
Feels in control, rarely experiences power struggles with others
Able to maturely address and handle issues as they arise
Contributes to respectful environment for others to express themselves
No stress-related health issues

Examples: "I would love to volunteer for the event but I don't have extra time right now."
"I make it a policy to never lend money to friends or family."
"I see that you are angry with me because you think I don't do my fair share. Here is why I see this differently than you."

Assertive Communication Concepts

1) Being assertive does not involve hurting the other person's feelings. The goal is to share information in a respectful manner.

2) Assertive communication seeks to equalize the balance of power, not win the fight by putting down another person or by manipulating another person's emotions.

3) Assertive communication involves expressing your legitimate rights as an individual. You have a *right* to express your own wants, needs, feelings, and ideas in a respectful manner.

4) Other individuals have a right to respond to your assertive communication with their own wants, needs, feelings, and ideas. If we want to be heard, we must be willing to listen. Remember, the only person we can control is ourselves but we can try to influence others.

5) An assertive encounter with another individual may involve negotiating an agreeable compromise.

6) Assertive communication enhances relationships with others.

7) Assertive behavior involves not only *what* you say, but *how* you say it, including word choice, tone, and body language.

8) Assertive words accompanied by appropriate body language reduces the defensiveness in others and makes your communication more effective.

9) Assertive body language includes maintaining direct but not intense eye contact, maintaining a relaxed posture, refraining from crossed arms, speaking clearly and intelligibly, using a mature and confident tone of voice, refraining from baby talk and whining, and smiling and nodding along with the other person's conversation.

10) Assertive behavior and communication can become second nature with practice.

ASSERTIVENESS ASSESSMENT

Mark situations where you have difficulty being assertive. Then identify the level of difficulty you have, 1 being slightly difficult, 2 being difficult, 3 being very difficult.

WHEN	CHECK IF YES	1=SLIGHTLY DIFFICULT 2=DIFFICULT 3=VERY DIFFICULT
Asking for help		
Stating a difference		
Expressing negative emotions		
Expressing positive emotions		
Addressing uncooperative behavior from others		
Communicating annoyance		
Speaking in front of a group		
Protesting a deception or being cheated		
Saying no		
Responding to undeserved criticism		
Making requests of authority figures		
Negotiating		
Being in charge		
Asking for cooperation		
Proposing an idea		
Asking questions		
Asking for clarification		
Asking for service		
Asking someone on a date		
Asking for favors		

WHO	CHECK IF YES	1=SLIGHTLY DIFFICULT 2=DIFFICULT 3=VERY DIFFICULT
Spouse or partner		
Friends		
Acquaintances		
Stranger		
Employer		
Co-workers		
Classmates		
Sales people, clerks, hired help		
Parents		
Children		
Relatives		
More than two or three people in a group		

WHAT	CHECK IF YES	1=SLIGHTLY DIFFICULT 2=DIFFICULT 3=VERY DIFFICULT
More time with spouse or partner		
Disagreeing with someone		
Addressing passive-aggressive behavior		
Getting a job, asking for interviews or a raise		
Doing something new or different		
Doing things that are fun or relaxing		
Making a decision about a major purchase		
Getting time by yourself		
Initiating a sexual experience		
Being comfortable with strangers, acquaintances		
Being comfortable with supervisors and subordinates		

Next, identify areas that are most problematic for you. For any items marked a '3,' identify one example whereby you can be more assertive using healthy communication techniques.

IMPROVING ASSERTIVE COMMUNICATION WORKSHEET	
ITEMS MARKED '3'	**ASSERTIVE COMMUNICATION**
Example: WHO, mother	*When you joke with my husband about my cooking skills, I feel embarrassed and inadequate because I am insecure about being a new wife and mother. I would appreciate it if you would only make positive, supportive statements.*

HEALTHY COMMUNICATION EXERCISE

Begin using healthy communication skills by practicing five times. It is easiest to begin with issues that are relatively insignificant. Write down your five communications.

ITEM	HEALTHY COMMUNICATION STATEMENT
Examples:	*When you put the toilet paper under instead of over, I feel annoyed.* *When you interrupt me, I feel unheard and unimportant.*
1.	
2.	
3.	
4.	
5.	

HOMEWORK DAY 9

MOST PEOPLE DO NOT LISTEN WITH THE INTENT TO UNDERSTAND; THEY LISTEN WITH THE INTENT TO REPLY. – STEPHEN COVEY

1) Complete Assertiveness Assessment, Improving Assertive Communication Worksheet, Healthy Communication Exercise.

2) Identify daily gratitude.

3) Complete an ABC worksheet on any situation.

4) Make a commitment to complete Day 10.

BE PROUD OF WHAT YOU ARE ACCOMPLISHING!!!

DAY 10 PROBLEM-SOLVING

Today's Objective: 1) Learn healthy problem-solving concepts 2) Explore impact of ineffective problem-solving approaches on our well-being 3) Learn framework for effective problem-solving

In today's lesson, we will begin by exploring types of problem-solvers. There are generally three types of problem-solvers; the Thoughtful Planner, the Quick Fixer, and the Avoider. Let's explore each type:

The Thoughtful Planner: Thoughtful planners view difficult problems as an opportunity to improve their lives. They try to understand a problem by breaking it down and sorting it out. The positive and negative consequences of each option are considered and weighed before a decision is made. Thoughtful planners view emotions, even negative ones, as helpful in their effort to resolve a problem. They react to difficult problems in a thoughtful and plan-oriented manner, rather than trying to avoid or rush to judgement with a quick fix. They are open to change and are flexible about solutions.

Impact on well-being: Thoughtful planners generally experience lower levels of depression and anxiety, lower levels of frustration, are confident with their ability to navigate life, and are least likely to be overwhelmed by circumstances.

Avoider: Avoiders are nervous and unsure of themselves insofar as making decisions. They find problems upsetting and overwhelming. They freeze and are thereby unable to decide because they are terrified of the consequences of being stuck with a bad decision. When faced with problems, avoiders experience the urge to run away and evade. To escape conflict, they frequently avoid honest discussions, especially when their views differ from others.

Impact on well-being: Avoiders often experience higher levels of anxiety and depression. They have trouble navigating their way through life and frequently get stuck in unhealthy jobs, relationships, friendships, and living situations.

Quick Fixer: Quick fixers solve problems by choosing the first promising idea that comes to mind, which is similar to avoiding. To stop the negative feelings quickly, the fastest or easiest solution in chosen. They rush to judgement to escape the anxiety of delaying a decision. Expediency over quality is the quick fixer's mantra.

Impact on well-being: Because of their impulsive decision-making style and their inability to plan, quick fixers frequently face negative consequences for their decisions. These negative consequences often lead to depression.

You may have different problem-solving styles in different areas of your life. For example, when it comes to relationships, you may avoid difficult or painful conversations and ignore problematic behaviors. But, when it comes to your money, you may have your finances budgeted to the penny, research various investment options, and make careful choices about large purchases. At work, to be expedient, you may make decisions quickly and choose the first viable option without researching and pondering alternative options.

For example, you may have the following profile: Money – Thoughtful Planner

Relationships – Avoider

Work – Quick Fixer

Let's examine your problem-solving style in different areas of your life:

Intimate Relationships _____

Family _____

Friends _____

Work _____

Money _____

Self _____

What are your problem-solving strengths and weaknesses?

Using the information you identified in the previous section, think about how your various problem-solving styles are helpful or unhelpful. Where do your approaches cause problems in your life? See if you can identify your problem-solving strengths and weaknesses, including ideas to overcome your weaknesses (think about using Healthy Communication techniques learned in Day 9). A good rule of thumb for a problematic style is to recognize when you overreact and underreact, as both scenarios tend to result in residual problems.

Strengths:

Weaknesses:

Exercise: Think of a time in your life when you were faced with a problem. Describe the problem:

What problem-solving style did you employ?

What improvements, if any, could you have made?

How would the outcome have changed if you had used a different problem-solving style?

Remember, a good problem-solver uses a thoughtful planner approach to solving problems. They do not allow negative emotions to drive the decision-making process. Your problem-solving style is not a commentary on your worth as an individual. Rather, it is a behavioral repertoire that can be learned and reinforced with repeated use. Any weaknesses you identify are simply skills to be learned, practiced, and developed.

Next, we will learn a framework for making good, thoughtful decisions. Use the following worksheet to make better decisions. Remember, when identifying a problem behavior, it is something someone does or doesn't do, or says or doesn't say. Labeling, such as "My husband is selfish" is not a problem identification, it is a criticism. Focus on the behavior.

6-STEP PROBLEM-SOLVING EXAMPLE

1.) Define the Problem:
My ex-husband consistently brings the kids home late on Sunday evenings. As a result, they get to bed late and Monday mornings are difficult.

2.) Generate Alternative Solutions:
  a) *Talk to him.*
  b) *Give my ex-husband the cold shoulder so he knows I am irritated.*
  c) *I pick the kids up from his house at the designated time.*

3.) Evaluate the Alternatives (consider positive and negative consequences of each solution, where applicable):

SOLUTION	EVALUATION	
	PROS	**CONS**
a	*I have an opportunity to practice healthy communication.*	*I tried this, we argue, nothing changes.*
b	*I feel better in the moment because I feel like I am getting even.*	*I fail to address the issue in a meaningful way. I deteriorate relations with the father of my children.*
c	*I have more control over pick up time.*	*I have to do more driving which is unfair.*

4.) Select the Best Alternative: *C is the best alternative.*

5.) Put the Plan into Action: *I start picking the kids up from him at our scheduled time.*

6.) Evaluate the Results: *The kids are getting home on time, getting their baths and dinner. Monday mornings are much smoother. The unfairness of doing more driving is less frustrating than the aggravation of having them home late. I have more control over Sunday evenings and everyone is in a better mood on Monday morning.*

6-STEP PROBLEM-SOLVING WORKSHEET

1.) Define the Problem:

_____

2.) Generate Alternative Solutions:

    a) _____

    b) _____

    c) _____

3.) Evaluate the Alternatives (consider positive and negative consequences of each solution, where applicable):

SOLUTION	EVALUATION	
	PROS	**CONS**
a		
b		
c		

4.) Select the Best Alternative: _____

5.) Put the Plan into Action: _____

6.) Evaluate the Results:

_____

_____

_____

HOMEWORK DAY 10

QUOTE OF THE DAY:

IF YOU CAN FIND A PATH WITH NO OBSTACLES, IT PROBABLY DOESN'T LEAD ANYWHERE. – FRANK A. CLARK

1) Determine your problem-solving styles. Determine your problem-solving strengths and weaknesses. Complete the problem-solving exercise. Complete a 6-step problem-solving worksheet.

2) Identify daily gratitude.

3) Take a break from ABC worksheets.

4) Make a commitment to complete Day 11.

YOU'RE DOING IT!!!

DAY 11 ANXIETY

Today's Objective: 1) Learn the basic reasons why we experience anxiety 2) Learn the difference between the two distinct origins in the brain of the anxiety response 3) Learn the basics of exposure therapy to begin to extinguish the anxiety response

Anxiety disorders affect an estimated 40 million people in the U.S., or about 18% of the population. Anxiety develops from genetics, brain chemistry, inherent personality predispositions, family of origin experiences, and other significant life events.

Anxiety is an emotional response to a perceived threat, whether it originates from our thoughts or from an environmental stimulus. The perceived threat can originate from a physical threat, such as a poisonous snake, or a psychological threat, such as a cheating spouse. Anxiety frequency ranges from infrequent to constant and intensity ranges from mildly annoying to debilitating.

Most of us experience anxiety as a negative event and this perception increases anxiety's hold over us. If you begin to regard anxiety as an important warning system that alerts you to pay attention, anxiety can become a useful tool. Changing your perspective on anxiety will also help you gain control over it.

It is important to remember that anxiety has adaptive value. In the appropriate circumstance, cautious avoidance, heightened vigilance, and readiness to act improves survival. Problematic forms of anxiety, on the other hand, unnecessarily activate our threat defenses and harm-avoidance apparatus. These functions, once activated, effectively derail the cognitive resources we need for information processing and daily functioning.

A great example of using anxiety as a helpful tool is feeling nervous about an upcoming interview or test. Feeling nervous and anxious can be helpful in that it will cause us to pay attention to the task and nudge us to devote our time and energy to preparing for the upcoming event in an effort to do well. In fact, small to moderate levels of anxiety are shown to improve performance.

For those with crippling anxiety, beginning to understand how to treat it is crucial to learning to live well. Today's lesson is, at best, introductory. In short, conquering anxiety involves retraining the brain and this process takes time. This information confirms that people who struggle with anxiety cannot simply "just stop it."

Anxiety disorders fall into several categories and treatments may vary depending on the source and type of your anxiety. The categories of anxiety include generalized anxiety disorder ("GAD"), obsessive-compulsive disorder ("OCD"), post-traumatic disorder ("PTSD"), social anxiety, panic disorder, and specific phobias.

Understanding the origins of anxiety in the brain

Anxiety can originate in the brain in two ways. One way anxiety originates is in the cortex, or the grey matter portion of the brain, which is responsible for thinking, logic, reasoning, and language. Because this part of the brain is responsible for thinking, distorted thoughts originate in the cortex, which can generate anxiety.

For example, I may generate a thought distortion of "I think I left the front door unlocked and someone is going to rob me today while I'm at work." This thought can create a feeling of anxiety and panic. It may not be triggered by an environmental stimulus.

For those who have experienced difficult childhoods, as discussed on Day 5, Childhood Abuse, the damaged and broken belief systems created by childhood experiences can generate negative and distorted thought processes. Consequently, pathological forms of anxiety often manifest in survivors of abuse. For that reason, we further explored the beliefs that underlie enduring forms of anxiety on Day 6, Challenging Beliefs, and on Day 8, Patterns of Thinking.

The exercises learned on Day 1, ABC Worksheets, as well as the worksheets on Days 5, 6, and 8, are forms of Cognitive Behavioral Therapy ("CBT"), and are also effective treatments used to combat anxiety. As you practice ABC Worksheets, you should begin to notice a reduction in your anxiety responses. As your thoughts become less distorted and more realistic, your anxiety should improve. Today's lesson is another step in the direction of ridding yourself of this unwelcome companion, which has likely plagued many of us since childhood.

Another way that the brain generates an anxiety response is via the amygdala. Anxiety that is generated in the amygdala is better known as the "fight or flight" response. This type of anxiety is created from a danger message from the environment. The brain registers a threat of some sort in the environment and creates a fear response. For many, the threat in the environment is not actual, but rather, it is perceived.

To demonstrate this concept, consider an example. Suppose I am in my car at a traffic light and someone approaches my window with a gun and demands that I give him my car. He is wearing a specific cologne that I can smell, he has a goatee, and he is wearing a blue shirt with a superman logo.

During the traumatic event, our brain instantly employs its sophisticated survival mechanisms. Among other processes that occur, one important process our brain performs is the amygdala attaches fear to the event, which creates anxiety when the memory is subsequently recalled.

Triggers in the environment retrieve the memory, which is accompanied by the fear that was paired with memory. In the example above, the blue superman shirt may become a trigger. If I am walking down the aisle of a store and someone walks by with the same or similar shirt, the shirt may trigger the memory of the event together with the accompanying fear. This learned fear response presents as anxiety.

This type of anxiety is based in the amygdala. It is not generated by our thoughts alone, but by environmental stimuli. This type of anxiety can also be treated with CBT, but exposure therapy is also extremely effective. Let's take a look at exposure therapy.

How exposure therapy works

Exposure therapy is a rather simple concept, but is actually counter-intuitive. For those with various types of anxiety, avoidance of anxiety-producing situations seems logical. If I have anxiety in social situations, such as public speaking, my instinct is to avoid any situations, such as jobs, that require public speaking.

The problem with avoidance is that it perpetuates the disease state. Using the blue shirt example above, my instinct will be to avoid exposure to the shirt and to anything associated with that event. Suppose the event occurred at Main and First Street. That intersection will produce the same anxiety response and my instinct will be to avoid that area because my brain has labeled it as dangerous. Had the event occurred at Second and Fourth Street, my brain would identify that intersection as dangerous.

As I continue to avoid any stimulus that arouses the anxiety response, the threat is confirmed in the pathways in my brain. The avoidance process actually confirms that danger, thus making anxiety worse over time. So, if avoidance perpetuates the disease state, then we must stop avoiding to conquer the anxiety response.

By exposing our brains to anxiety producing situations that are not actually dangerous, our brains have an opportunity for new learning. The exposure process is crucial because those circuits in the brain that stored the memory and associated intense fear response must be activated in order for new learning to occur in the amygdala.

There are two ways to accomplish exposure therapy: flooding and systematic desensitization. Flooding involves direct, immediate exposure exercises. For example, using the blue shirt example above, sitting with a blue shirt with a superman logo every day for 45 minutes at a time is an example of flooding. Each day that the brain is exposed to the shirt and nothing dangerous happens, the anxiety response becomes decreasingly intense and ultimately extinguishes in favor of new learning.

For some, direct exposure is too anxiety-producing to be helpful or productive. A great example is veterans going to the big box store. Those stores represent too much chaos and unpredictability to tolerate and their instinct is to flee. In these kinds of situations, we use systematic desensitization, which allows a stepwise approach to the feared stimulus.

An example of systematic desensitization might look like this: Step 1: driving by the big box store daily until there is no anxiety; Step 2: pulling into the parking lot daily until there is no anxiety; Step 3: sitting in the parking spot at the big box store daily until there is no anxiety; Step 4: parking and walking up to the front doors daily until there is no anxiety; Step 5: walking into the entrance daily until there is no anxiety; Step 6: walking into the store and walking around the front half of the store daily until there is no anxiety; Step 7: walking around the entire store daily until there is no anxiety.

Use the following worksheets to begin practicing exposure therapy. When designing your exercise, determine first whether to use the flooding worksheet or whether it is best to utilize the systematic desensitization worksheet.

During the exercise, it is crucial to stick with the exercise and refrain from leaving. Fleeing the exercise confirms the danger of the situation to the brain. The amygdala needs to learn new information and needs to learn that escape is not necessary.

Set yourself up for success. Choose an exercise, if possible, that you can complete at home. Looking at images on the internet is a great way to design exposure exercises. For example, a fear of spiders may involve looking at images of arachnids.

It is also important to refrain from using any anxiety reducing medications, in particular, benzodiazepines. These medications inhibit the activation of the amygdala, which is a necessary process for new learning to occur. Keep in mind, we must activate the fear response in order to extinguish it.

To conduct the exercise, choose a situation that causes some significant discomfort, but not complete panic. It is important to choose an exercise that you will be able to complete. Create a measurement scale that spans from 0 to 100. You will remain with the exercise for approximately 45 minutes, or until your anxiety subsides by at least half.

For example, if you begin looking at images of arachnids and you measure your anxiety at a 50, stay with the exercise until your anxiety measures 25. During the exercise, your anxiety may spike. Measure your peak anxiety if you experience an increase.

If your anxiety has not subsided sufficiently after 45 minutes, add 10 minute increments until it subsides. Do not use distraction techniques such as listening to music or watching television. Distractions interfere with new learning.

FLOODING EXPOSURE EXERCISE

Situation _____

Time: 45 minutes

DATE	BEGINNING 0 - 100	PEAK 0 - 100	FINAL 0 - 100

SYSTEMATIC DESENSITIZATION EXAMPLE

STEP	SITUATION	DATE	BEGINNING	PEAK	FINAL
1	Drive by the big box store	1/15	80	85	45
		1/16	80	80	40
		1/17	75	85	40
		1/18	75	80	35
2	Pull into the parking lot at the big box store	1/19	85	85	40
		1/21	75	75	40
		1/22	70	70	35
		1/23	70	70	35
3	Sitting in a parking spot at the big box store	1/24	75	75	35
		1/25	70	70	35
		1/26	60	65	30
		1/27	60	60	30
4	Parking and walking to the front doors of the big box store	1/29	75	80	40
		1/30	70	75	35
		1/31	60	60	30
		2/1	55	60	30
5	Walking into the entrance at the big box store	2/2	70	80	35
		2/4	60	60	30
		2/5	60	60	30
		2/7	55	60	25
6	Walking into the store and walking around the front half	2/8	60	70	30
		2/9	55	60	25
		2/11	50	60	25
		2/12	40	50	25
7	Walking around the entire store	2/14	50	70	25
		2/15	50	60	25
		2/16	40	40	20
		2/17	30	40	15

SYSTEMATIC DESENSITIZATION

STEP	SITUATION	DATE	BEGINNING	PEAK	FINAL
1					
2					
3					
4					
5					
6					
7					

HOMEWORK DAY 11

NEVER BE AFRAID TO TRY SOMETHING NEW. REMEMBER,
AMATEURS BUILT THE ARK, PROFESSIONALS BUILT THE TITANIC.
– LOUIS MENAND

1) Set up and begin an exposure therapy exercise using the flooding or the systematic desensitization worksheet.

2) Identify daily gratitude.

3) Complete an ABC worksheet on a situation that produces anxiety.

4) Make a commitment to complete Day 12.

GREAT WORK! TAKE A MOMENT TO REFLECT ON YOUR PROGRESS!!!

DAY 12 NEEDS

Today's Objective: 1) Learn about human needs 2) Begin the process of identifying individual needs 3) Begin the process of having your needs met

Today we will explore the concept of needs. Many people are out of touch with their needs; many are unaware they have needs at all. For survivors of child abuse, the mere concept of HAVING needs can induce a shame response. The insidious nature of abuse is such that it facilitates the child's denial of their own needs. The child then carries this pattern of need-denial into adulthood.

For children in the midst of abuse, the experiences of abuse communicate an unspoken message that the child does not deserve to have their needs met, or worse, does not deserve to have needs *at all*. In a frantic effort to remain connected to the abuser, the child will also try to normalize and thereby justify the abuser's behavior. To reconcile the conflict between their own needs and the abuser's desires/behaviors, the child will disconnect from themselves. For those exposed to significant and/or prolonged abuse, the child morphs into an existence reduced to mere survival. Many of the joyful memories of childhood are eclipsed and replaced by the presence of a vigilant fight-or-flight/reactive-reality.

In today's lesson, as we begin the process of naming and exploring needs, we will make connections to worthiness. Many individuals struggle with feelings of worthlessness which, in turn, fuel depression and anxiety.

On Day 5, Childhood Abuse, we began to identify negative beliefs. Knowing that we all have needs as human beings and identifying those needs, helps us begin to understand that we are all inherently, unconditionally worthy of love and acceptance.

First, let's begin by examining the biologically-based core needs we all share.

Satisfaction of core needs is universal and necessary for healthy human development. Meeting our core needs in infancy and childhood is the fundamental responsibility of our primary caregivers.

For survivors of child abuse, the nature of developmental trauma is such that it denies us some or all of our biologically-based core needs. When this happens, we fail to develop a solid foundation from which to confidently and competently grow and engage the world.

Let's take a look at the five core needs and what happens to us when they are not met.

The five core needs that are crucial and foundational for healthy human development include the need for connection, attunement, trust, autonomy, and love-sexuality.

The need for connection is identified as the ability to understand our bodies and our emotions, as well as connect and bond with others.

The need for attunement is the need for awareness of our own needs and emotions, and to identify, request, and receive nurturance from others.

The need for trust includes the ability to develop healthy dependence on others, as well as the capacity for interdependence.

The need for autonomy includes the identification and establishment of healthy boundaries, and the ability to express ourselves without negative consequence.

The need for love-sexuality includes the ability to love others without fear and to (later) establish a healthy sexual relationship with others.

It is self-evident that infants are incapable of meeting these need for themselves and they are therefore placed in a vulnerable position to their caregivers. Improper caregiving and abuse places children at risk of developing inadequate self-images, low self-esteem, and insufficient self-regulation.

When core needs are not met in childhood, unhealthy adaptive strategies are immobilized in an effort to manage the pain and dysregulation associated with abuse. These adaptations, in favor of survival, that begin in infancy carry into adulthood and present as psychological and physiological dysfunction.

When the need for connection is not met, it is our survival instinct to numb and we thereby become disconnected from our physical bodies and our emotions. It is then a natural outgrowth that we have difficulty attaching to others.

When the need for attunement is not met, we fail to develop an ability to identify our needs. When we grow up in an environment that denies our needs, we learn to deny them as well. The net result is that we either cannot identify our needs or, when we can, we feel unworthy of asserting them or having them met.

When our need for trust is not met, we will learn to depend only on ourselves and we will develop a need to be in control. When we are not in control we will often feel out of control. Unfortunately, our need to control often extends to others and ultimately destroys the intimacy we desire.

When our need for autonomy is not met, we will develop a fear of setting boundaries, a fear of demonstrating independence, or an inability to say 'no.' Failing to assert ourselves, we often feel mistreated or taken advantage of after-the-fact, which leads to resentment.

When our need for love-sexuality is not met, we will develop unhealthy and inappropriate sexual boundaries, as well as a superficial self-esteem based on physical appearance and/or productivity.

Many individuals experience some variation of deficiency in the attainment of these five core needs and thus develop unhealthy adaptations as a means of survival. What was adaptive, at the time, becomes maladaptive over time.

For those who are unaware of their needs, life becomes the equivalent of taking a journey with no roadmap or destination. Life is reduced to a confusing litany of stop and go activities without any clear direction or purpose. And without direction and purpose, life has no meaning. Many people report experiencing this as feeling adrift.

Today's lesson is only a preliminary start to identifying and meeting our own needs.

For today's worksheet, begin by using the List of Needs to identify a need. Use the worksheet to identify the need in the 'Need' column. In the 'Obstacle' column, identify one obstacle that you put in your own way that keeps you from having that need met (by yourself or by others). Think of the adaptive styles. In the last column, 'Step,' identify one step, however small, that you can take to remove the obstacle in favor of pursuing a direction that culminates in having your needs met.

LIST OF NEEDS

Connection
Acceptance
Affection
Appreciation
Belonging
Cooperation
Communication
Closeness
Community
Companionship
Compassion
Consideration
Consistency
Empathy
Inclusion
Intimacy
Love
Nurturing
Respect/Self-Respect
Safety
Security
Stability
Support
To Know and Be Known
To Understand and Be Understood
Trust
Warmth
Physical Well-Being
Sexual Expression
Touch
Safe Shelter
Honesty
Authenticity
Integrity

Freedom
Independence
Spontaneity
Meaning
Awareness
Celebration of Life
Challenge
Clarity
Competence
Consciousness
Contribution
Creativity
Discovery
Efficacy
Effectiveness
Growth
Hope
Learning
Participation
Purpose
Self-Expression
Stimulation
To Matter
Choice
Autonomy
Order
Inspiration
Harmony
Equality
Beauty
Peace
Humor
Joy
Play

NEED	OBSTACLE	STEP
Example: *Growth*	*Fear of failure. I have stayed in the same job and do not try new activities. I stay in the same relationships and keep the same friends. I am afraid to go back to school.*	*Recognize my fear and begin researching school programs for nursing.*

HOMEWORK DAY 12

1) Complete Needs worksheet.

2) Identify daily gratitude.

3) Conduct exposure therapy or complete an ABC worksheet on any situation.

4) Make a commitment to complete Day 13.

AWESOME WORK!!!

DAY 13 WHAT DO I...

Today's Objective: Continue to identify and refine our sense of self

In yesterday's lesson, we began the process of identifying our own needs. Today's lesson will expand on yesterday's concept of self-identification to define and refine a clearer sense of who we are as a person. This, and several lessons in this book, assist with the process of self-discovery.

One of the fascinating aspects of human nature, which makes the field of mental health so fascinating, is that we are all unique – we are all one of a kind. Unfortunately, in the throes of depression, we may not see ourselves as special, deserving, or worthy. Depression has a way of robbing us of the things that matter most – including the ability to value ourselves.

For today's lesson, begin by using the worksheet entitled 'What Do I' to further develop your sense of self. To get started, use the List of Values to begin identifying what makes you uniquely you. Complete the rest of the worksheet in a similar fashion. Finally, answer the questions for further self-discovery.

WHAT DO I:	
VALUE	
HATE	
JUDGE	
HONOR	
DESIRE	
COMMIT TO	
LOVE	
HOPE FOR	
BELIEVE IN	
TRUST	

LIST OF VALUES				
Acceptance	Courtesy	Hard Work	Patience	Restraint
Accomplishment	Creativity	Harmony	Patriotism	Results
Accountability	Credibility	Health	Perfection	Reverence
Accuracy	Curiosity	Heroism	Performance	Risk
Achievement	Dedication	Holiness	Perseverance	Rule of Law
Adaptability	Dependability	Honesty	Persistence	Sacrifice
Adventure	Determination	Honor	Personal Growth	Safety
Altruism	Devotion	Hope	Persuasiveness	Security
Ambition	Diligence	Humbleness	Philanthropy	Self-Awareness
Assertiveness	Directness	Humility	Play	Self-Motivation
Belonging	Diversity	Humor	Pleasantness	Self-Control
Bravery	Drive	Imagination	Poise	Self-Reliance
Candor	Education	Individuality	Popularity	Sense of Humor
Capability	Effectiveness	Innovation	Positivity	Service to Others
Change	Efficiency	Integrity	Power	Silliness
Character	Empathy	Intelligence	Pragmatic	Simplicity
Citizenship	Engagement	Joy	Precision	Sincerity
Cleanliness	Enthusiasm	Justice	Preparedness	Spontaneity
Collaboration	Equality	Kindness	Privacy	Stewardship
Commitment	Excellence	Knowledge	Professionalism	Strength
Communication	Experience	Leadership	Prosperity	Structure
Compassion	Expertise	Loyalty	Punctuality	Success
Competence	Exploration	Mastery	Rational	Support
Competition	Faith	Maturity	Realistic	Sympathy
Composure	Family	Moderation	Reason	Tolerance
Confidence	Fidelity	Motivation	Recognition	Tradition
Confidentiality	Fitness	Obedience	Recreation	Tranquility
Connection	Flexibility	Open-Mindedness	Relaxation	Transparency
Consistency	Freedom	Openness	Reliability	Truth
Contentment	Generosity	Optimism	Resilience	Understanding
Control	Giving	Order	Resourcefulness	Uniqueness
Conviction	Gratitude	Organization	Respect	Valor
Cooperation	Growth	Originality	Responsiveness	Work/Life Balance
Courage	Happiness	Passion	Rest	

Next, answer the following questions:

What are you pretending not to know?

Why don't you do the things you know you should be doing?

Are you being true to your values?

What don't you know that you wish you could learn?

Are your 'shoulds' getting in the way of your happiness?

If you achieved all of your life's goals, how would you feel? How can you feel that along the way?

What did you learn today?

What made you laugh today?

If you weren't scared what would you do?

If you were dying, would you change what you worry about?

Can you determine when you should be focused on today or tomorrow?

What keeps you from trying? What would happen if you tried to pursue something you are afraid of?

What or who did you make better today?

What do you want your life to be in 5 years?

What can you do today to improve?

What is the one most important thing to get done today/this week/this month/this year?

Today:

Week:

Month:

Year:

If you could wave a magic want and do anything, what would happen?

What qualities do your role models have?

HOMEWORK DAY 13

THE HIGHER WE SOAR, THE SMALLER WE APPEAR TO THOSE WHO CANNOT FLY. – FRIEDRICH NIETZSCHE

1) Complete What Do I worksheet and answer questions.

2) Identify daily gratitude.

3) Conduct exposure therapy and take a break from ABC worksheets.

4) Make a commitment to complete Day 14.

GOOD JOB TODAY! YOU CAN DO THIS!!!

DAY 14 POSITIVE QUALITIES

Today's Objective: 1) Identify positive qualities, gifts, and talents you possess 2) Begin to view yourself in a positive way

In today's lesson, you will begin (perhaps for the first time) to speak in a kind way to yourself. For many people, negative self-talk is a tape that involuntarily runs in the background on a constant basis. This negative self-talk affects your mood and influences your behavior.

It is impossible to develop solid, positive self-esteem with a negative view of yourself. Many people struggle with low self-esteem and recognize the problem but feel powerless to change it.

Good self-esteem combined with the ability to identify your own positive qualities will enable you to experience greater fulfillment in life.

We all have positive qualities and we all have inherent value as individuals. Viewing yourself in a positive light, coupled with possessing a solid grounding in your own personal values (identified in yesterday's lesson), will guide positive behavior because the combination helps solidify your personal code of conduct. Living and behaving congruently with your personal code of conduct contributes to fulfillment and satisfaction in life.

In other words, when the way we behave honors and reflects those things we hold dear, we live with a greater sense of purpose and contentment.

For today's lesson, use the following worksheet to begin to identify and name your positive qualities. Use the word list to pinpoint those qualities and write them in the left-hand column of the worksheet.

In order to possess the quality, you do not need to exhibit it 100% of the time. For example, you can write 'generous' as a quality even if you do not give away everything you own.

Next to the quality you identify, use a specific example to solidify the belief. Then take a moment to appreciate the positive emotional experience that arises from this recognition.

POSITIVE QUALITIES

Accepting	Diplomatic	Hopeful	Outgoing	Results-oriented
Adaptable	Direct	Humorous	Particular	Self-reliant
Ambitious	Dynamic	Imaginative	Patient	Sensible
Appreciative	Eager	Independent	Perceptive	Sensitive
Assertive	Easy-going	Industrious	Personable	Sincere
Balanced	Eclectic	Informal	Persuasive	Skilled
Capable	Emotional	Insightful	Pleasant	Sociable
Caring	Empathetic	Intelligent	Positive	Solid
Cautious	Enthusiastic	Interesting	Powerful	Spunky
Charming	Entrepreneurial	Inventive	Practical	Stable
Cheerful	Exciting	Kind	Precise	Strong
Clever	Faithful	Knowledgeable	Proactive	Tactful
Communicative	Fast	Leader	Productive	Talented
Compassionate	Flexible	Literate	Professional	Tenacious
Competent	Focused	Logical	Progressive	Thorough
Competitive	Forgiving	Loving	Punctual	Thoughtful
Confident	Free-spirited	Methodical	Quick	Traditional
Conscientious	Friendly	Modest	Quirky	Trustworthy
Consistent	Generous	Neat	Rational	Unconventional
Cooperative	Gentle	Non-judgmental	Rebellious	Understanding
Courageous	Genuine	Observant	Reliable	Unique
Curious	Good Listener	Open-minded	Reserved	Versatile
Dependable	Grateful	Optimistic	Resilient	Warm
Determined	Helpful	Organized	Respectful	Wise
Devoted	Honest	Original	Responsible	Witty

QUALITY	EXAMPLE

HOMEWORK DAY 14

1) Complete the Positive Qualities worksheet with supporting examples.

2) Identify daily gratitude.

3) Conduct exposure therapy and complete an ABC worksheet on any situation.

4) Make a commitment to complete Day 15.

YOU GOT THIS!!!

DAY 15 ATTACHMENTS

Today's Objective: 1) Learn about attachment 2) Learn about the impact of attachment on relationships 3) Learn how to begin to heal and improve attachment-related issues

What is attachment and why is it important?

In today's lesson, we will learn about the concepts and mechanisms of attachment to more thoroughly understand our functioning, especially as it relates to our relationship behaviors and our overall mental health.

Attachment is the bonding process that begins at birth between an infant and a primary caregiver whereby the needs of the infant are met. This process facilitates emotional, cognitive, neurological, and social development. In the most basic sense, attachment is (optimally) that safe and secure physical and emotional habitat, which fosters growth and confidence. Consequently, our attachment determines the way will engage and interact with the world around us.

A child's natural instinct from birth is to use involuntary responses to send a signal to the caregiver, such as crying. A child who receives an appropriate response from his/her caregiver learns that others are accessible, attentive, and can therefore be trusted. A child who grows up in this environment forms a secure attachment and feels loved, nurtured, and secure. Children with secure attachments can engage and interact with the world with trust and confidence.

For children, attachment is about survival. Consequently, children who do not experience attuned caregiving develop survival adaptations. A word about Maslow's hierarchy of needs is crucial to understanding the evolution that takes place both with, and without, proper caregiving.

Maslow developed a theory of human motivation over 75 years ago and later expanded his observations to explain the innate curiosity of humans. Maslow described a hierarchical system through which human motivations generally progress. The need to satisfy physiological needs for survival is the most basic of human needs, following by the need for safety. What is central about Maslow's theory to understanding attachment is that until basic needs are met, humans do not pursue the satisfaction of higher order needs such as love and belonging, esteem, and ultimately self-actualization (see diagram). Consequently, children without proper caregiving, whose attachments are compromised, often remain in a perpetual cycle aimed at satisfying only their basic human needs.

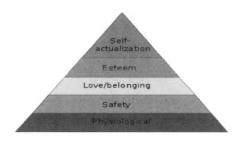

When an unstable foundation/attachment is formed, individuals often experience anxiety, depression, despair, and sometimes potentially permanent attachment disorders. Observing the behavioral differences of feral cats versus houses cats/pets is an excellent example of this distinction. Feral cats, keen on survival, interact with their environments with extreme caution and often react quickly and socially retreat. They do not enjoy the leisurely life of sleeping soundly (for hours), exploring without fear, and immersing themselves in an environment where they can rely upon having their physiological needs met and receiving affection (only on their terms, of course). Our survival adaptations are similar in that we are more guarded about our environment, less trusting that people are safe or reliable, and therefore less engaging in both physical and social/emotional environments. Consequently, this adaptation, in humans and animals, predicts/dictates the behavioral sequence that follows.

It is understandable then that the manner in which a child attaches to a caregiver has a profound impact on personality development as well as the child's sense of security. As children experience attachment patterns throughout childhood, working models for relationships are formed in the brain. These patterns of beliefs, emotional responses, and behavioral sequences continue into adulthood. Undisputedly, the quality of early attachment influences an individual's future ability to form attachments to others.

These early relationships play a significant role in the formulation of intimate relationship patterns that are experienced in adulthood. These experiences also play a substantial role in other life domains such as how we manage loss or navigate traumatic experiences.

Adult intimate relationships share the following similarities with infant-caregiver relationships:

- Mutual feelings of attraction and enchantment
- A sense of safety when near an attachment figure
- The ability to experience physical closeness that is reciprocal
- Insecurity when the attachment figure is not available
- Ability to explore the world together
- Mirroring facial and physical movement
- Use of baby talk

Attachment experiences result in three basic types of attachment styles in adult relationships: anxious, avoidant, and secure. Each attachment pattern has a predictable emotional and behavioral sequence.

An anxious attachment style is characterized by worry about a partner's love and commitment, worry that the partner is not reliable, a need for accessibility and reassurance, and a tendency to take things personally. Individuals with an anxious attachment style want closeness and intimacy, but are hypersensitive to signs of rejection.

An avoidant attachment style is characterized by valuing independence and freedom over the connectedness of a relationship, difficulty sharing feelings, and blaming behaviors. Individuals with an avoidant attachment style prefer not to rely on others, send mixed signals in relationships, and tend to miss nonverbal signals from their partners (because of their lack of connectedness).

A secure attachment style is marked by a balance between the extremes of anxious and avoidant attachment styles. A secure person exhibits few emotional difficulties, generally feels safe and comfortable with intimacy, and does not exhibit undue stress over the relationship. These individuals experience low anxiety in relationships, are consistent and reliable, and are comfortable with closeness and commitment. Secure partners are the most stable partners and two secure partners are recognizable by a generally solid relationship. In other words, the stronger the foundation upon which you build a relationship, the stronger the relationship.

Now let's determine your attachment style. Answer the questions honestly in order to gain the most accurate picture of your style. Having an honest assessment of your style is important in order to facilitate healthier relationships. The following questionnaire is from *Attached. The New Science of Adult Attachment and How It Can Help You Find – and Keep – Love* written by Levine and Heller, 2010.

Mark the box of the statements that are TRUE for you. If the statement is not true for you, do not mark the box.

	TRUE		
	A	**B**	**C**
I often worry that my partner will stop loving me.	☐		
I find it easy to be affectionate with my partner.		☐	
I fear that once someone gets to know the real me, s/he won't like who I am.	☐		
I find that I bounce back quickly after a breakup. It's weird how I can just put someone out of my mind.			☐
When I'm not involved in a relationship, I feel somewhat anxious and incomplete.	☐		
I find it difficult to emotionally support my partner when s/he is feeling down.			☐
When my partner is away, I'm afraid that s/he might become interested in someone else.	☐		
I feel comfortable depending on romantic partners.		☐	
My independence is more important to me than my relationships.			☐
I prefer not to share my innermost feelings with my partner.			☐
When I show my partner how I feel, I'm afraid s/he will not feel the same about me.	☐		
I am generally satisfied with my romantic relationships.		☐	
I don't feel the need to act out much in my romantic relationships.		☐	
I think about my relationships a lot.	☐		
I find it difficult to depend on romantic partners.			☐
I tend to get very quickly attached to a romantic partner.	☐		
I have little difficulty expressing my needs and wants to my partner.		☐	
I sometimes feel angry or annoyed with my partner without knowing why.			☐

	TRUE		
	A	**B**	**C**
I am very sensitive to my partner's moods.	☐		
I believe most people are essentially honest and dependable.		☐	
I prefer casual sex with uncommitted partners to intimate sex with one person.			☐
I'm comfortable sharing my personal thoughts and feelings with my partner.		☐	
I worry that if my partner leaves me I might never find someone else.	☐		
It makes me nervous when my partner gets too close.			☐
During a conflict, I tend to impulsively do or say things I later regret, rather than be able to reason about things.	☐		
An argument with my partner doesn't usually cause me to question our entire relationship.		☐	
My partners often want me to be more intimate than I feel comfortable being.			☐
I worry that I'm not attractive enough.	☐		
Sometimes people see me as boring because I create little drama in relationships.		☐	
I miss my partner when we're apart, but then when we're together, I feel the need to escape.			☐
When I disagree with someone, I feel comfortable expressing my opinions.		☐	
I hate feeling that other people depend on me.			☐
If I notice that someone I'm interested in is checking out other people, I don't let it faze me. I might feel a pang of jealousy, but it's fleeting.		☐	
If I notice that someone I'm interested in is checking out other people, I feel relieved – it means s/he's not looking to make things exclusive.			☐
If I notice that someone I'm interested in is checking out other people, it makes me feel depressed.	☐		
If someone I've been dating begins to act cold and distant, I may wonder what's happened, but I'll know it's probably not about me.		☐	
If someone I've been dating begins to act cold and distant, I'll probably be indifferent; I might even be relieved.			☐

	TRUE		
	A	**B**	**C**
If someone I've been dating begins to act cold and distant, I'll worry that I've done something wrong.	☐		
If my partner was to break up with me, I'd try my best to show him/her what s/he is missing (a little jealousy can't hurt).	☐		
If someone I've been dating for several months tells me s/he wants to stop seeing me, I'd feel hurt at first, but I'd get over it.		☐	
Sometimes when I get what I want in a relationship, I'm not sure what I want anymore.			☐
I won't have much of a problem staying in touch with my ex (strictly platonic) – after all, we have a lot in common.		☐	

Total A column _____

Total B column _____

Total C column _____

Identify your highest score. The items in the A column represent the anxious attachment style, column B represent the secure style, and column C represent the avoidant style.

If you have difficulty identifying your style, the book or a qualified therapist will helpful.

Now that you have identified your style, let's look at some common behaviors that negatively affect relationships.

Anxious attachment style behaviors:

- Obsessive thoughts about your partner, especially in their absence.
- Ignoring or rationalizing negative traits, qualities, and behaviors in your partner.
- Idealizing your partner.
- Believing your partner is the only one for you.
- Believing and expecting your partner will change.
- Reduced anxiety when your partner is physically close.
- Using hostility and manipulation in order to arouse an emotional response.
- Sensitivity to perceived rejection.
- Excessive need for reassuring statements.

Becoming aware of the anxious attachment style is the first step to becoming more secure in your attachments. Knowing that there is a reason for your anxious feelings that has to do with your attachment system and perhaps not the relationship is very empowering because now you have more control over your emotions. The use of ABC worksheets to manage emotional and behavioral responses is extremely helpful, along with recognizing catastrophic thought patterns and healthy communication skills to express your feelings and needs.

Avoidant attachment style behaviors:

- Avoiding commitment but remain in a relationship.
- Becoming annoyed by their partner, intolerance for imperfections.
- Maintaining a longing for former partners.
- Exhibiting flirting behaviors, which is a passive-aggressive way to generate insecurity in a partner.
- Holding back terms of endearment, refrain from saying 'I love you' but send signals of love.
- Pulling back after intimacy.
- Becoming involved with married partners.
- Keeping secrets.
- Remaining physically distant, lack of affection and sexual activity, refrain from sharing a bed.

Just as with the anxious attachment style, becoming aware of avoidant tendencies is the first step in moving towards more secure attachments. Using ABC worksheets, healthy communication skills, becoming aware of your own needs, and identifying gratitude regarding the relationship are also great starts for healthier, more stable, calmer relationships.

Answer the following questions to further work through anxious and avoidant attachment styles.

1) What situations and relationship dynamics are most likely to trigger your anxiety or avoidant reactions?

2) What is the effect on your relationship of these reactions?

3) What are your underlying fears in the situation (see Day 3, Fears)?

4) What secure attachment behaviors would have had a more positive effect on the situation and the relationship?

5) What would your partner's reaction to more secure behaviors be?

HOMEWORK DAY 15

NEVER WASTE YOUR FEELINGS ON PEOPLE WHO DON'T VALUE THEM. – ARFA MALIK

1) Complete attachment questions.

2) Identify daily gratitude.

3) Conduct exposure therapy and take a break from ABC worksheets.

4) Make a commitment to complete Day 16.

HALF WAY THERE!!!

DAY 16 EXPECTATIONS

Today's Objective 1) Learn different types of expectations 2) Learn how expectations interfere with optimal functioning

Many people mistakenly believe the solution to disappointment is to avoid having expectations of anyone. There are many quotes that appear to support this theory such as, "The best way to avoid disappointment is to not expect anything from anyone." Truthfully, these statements are depressing, they are unrealistic, and they further the divide between us.

Emotional connectivity is a beautiful part of the human experience. Furthermore, bonding, which lays the groundwork for emotional connectivity, cannot occur without some level of expectation involving loyalty, behavioral accountability, and commitment. In other words, we are right to expect our partner to honor the pillars of a healthy relationship.

Realistic expectations for ourselves and others have a positive, almost profound, impact on both functioning and achievement. In a 1960s Harvard research study, public elementary school teachers were falsely informed that certain students were gifted. As a result, teachers' expectations of these students increased, as did student performance in the classroom and on standardized tests. This phenomenon is why our own internal belief system is central to our performance and happiness. That concept is especially true because, in many ways, we spend our lives confirming what we already believe.

When we believe in ourselves, we actually utilize more of our brainpower and exhibit better problem-solving skills. Believing in yourself is crucial in terms of achievement because we need the ability to overcome obstacles and to look at problems from different points of view. Having expectations of ourselves lays the groundwork for achievement.

However, it is important to keep those expectations reasonable. There is nothing wrong with lofty goals, as long as they are attainable. For example, believing I am going to be the next American Idol winner is unrealistic – it is not going to happen. All the voice lessons in the world will not land me in the winner's circle! Believing this will happen will only lead to disappointment and heartache.

Some expectations are grounded in reason and experience. I have an expectation that my spouse will be faithful to me. I also have an expectation that my employer will pay me for work I perform. Those expectations are reasonable because they approximate what is likely to happen, and they properly consider my prior experiences.

Sometimes our intense desire for something that is not likely to occur morphs into an expectation that it will. Unfortunately, unreasonable expectations actually interfere with our lives and our relationships. They set us up for hurt and disappointment. In today's lesson, we will examine some that commonly occur, then we will use a worksheet to begin to address them.

Common expectations that actually set us up for disappointment

1) **Life should be fair.** "Life's not fair" is a maxim for a reason. But these lessons of fairness are hardwired in our brains. They are a large part of childhood experiences and part of the way our brains make sense of the world around us. Try giving a child a box of new crayons and another child one broken orange crayon, tell them to draw a picture, and see what happens. Unfortunately, the adult world does not involve convincing another child to share their box of crayons. Using your cognitive skills and utilizing unfair experiences as learning opportunities are crucial to managing life's disparities and disappointments.

2) **Opportunities will fall into my lap.** Although there are times in life when good things just spontaneously happen, we create most (if not all) of our opportunity through hard work. So, what happens when hard work does not pan out? Sometimes a new relationship is not just around the corner. Sometimes the promotion we deserve does not materialize. Sometimes getting a degree does not translate into a job. A combination of hard work and lessons learned from situations that do not work out as we hoped teaches us the importance of moving past a wrongly held expectation.

3) **Everyone should like me.** Most people have difficulty accepting that they are not liked by someone. It is human nature to want to be liked and this desire originates from our survival instincts wherein we need to be accepted/included in a group to increase our chances of continued existence. This dynamic applies to a psychological situation as much as it applies to a physical survival scenario – our brains do not distinguish between the two. A great solution to this expectation, which is a major source of anxiety for people, is to focus instead on earning respect and trust. Another solution is to recognize that you do not like everyone you meet. Sometimes we do not like people because they are different from us. And sometimes we do not even know why we do not like someone. Accepting that others can have these same experiences with us helps us shed this unrealistic expectation. It is both healthy and natural to desire the companionship of some and avoid the companionship of others. Since it is a natural process, it is best not to take it personally.

4) **People should agree with me.** From a young age, we are primed to believe there are winners and losers and that we are either right or we are wrong. When we are confronted with an opinion that differs from ours, we instinctually respond as if we are losing or failing. For that reason (among others), it is hard for many people to accept input from others. That concept is especially true when we feel knowledgeable and competent in certain areas of our life. However, if everyone always agreed with us then we would never gain new knowledge. The most difficult aspect of gaining that knowledge involves listening to the perspective of another versus defending our own position. Focusing on gaining a new perspective from a different vantage point enhances our understanding of ourselves and others. When we are comfortable with who we are, we can be enlightened, as opposed to threatened, by a different point of view. Besides, when we stop learning, we stop growing.

5) **People should know what I mean.** This expectation can be a bit subtle at times because others may not ask you for clarification if they do not understand. Our intentions can be irrelevant when we hurt others (we will discuss this concept on Day 20, Repairing Wounds). Other people cannot read your mind and, remember, others have different perspectives, beliefs, and histories. The message you intend may be very different from what someone else hears. Being clear and thorough with your communications minimizes misunderstandings and expectations. Confirming that the recipient understood your message as intended goes a long way to avoiding misunderstandings and the hurt feelings that result.

6) **I'm going to fail.** Sometimes, as a way to protect ourselves from disappointment, we prepare ourselves for failure. Unfortunately, when we tell ourselves we are going to fail before we even try, it dampens our willingness to attempt what we desire, and it increases the likelihood that we will quit at the first sign of resistance. In reality, when we tell ourselves we will fail, we set ourselves up for failure. Remember, we spend much of our lives confirming what we already believe.

7) **I will be happy once I get (fill in material thing).** Ask yourself this question: If I am not happy with what I have, what makes me think I will be happy with more? The joy of getting something new and shiny is fleeting and often anticlimactic/empty. Many times, it does not satiate our desire, it intensifies it. New things can be intoxicating, especially with the variety of material things available and the ease of making purchases. Focus instead on appreciating what you have (daily gratitude!) and identifying any emotional voids the material things are filling.

8) **I can change him/her.** Many people, especially women, get into relationships with an expectation that the other person will change once the person is "fixed." There is an often-quoted sentiment that women get into relationships hoping that men will change, and men get into relationships hoping that women won't change. We can certainly influence others, in an assortment of ways, including healthy communication, but we do not have the ability to morph people into what we want or need them to be. Nor should we. Everyone acts from their own needs and motivations and these are very difficult to change. Think about changing yourself to suit someone else's needs and you will begin to see that others do not change to meet our needs. In fact, if we wish to be appreciated for who we are, we need to appreciate others for who they are, as well. And when we do that, they will appreciate us even more.

9) **Others should know "how I am."** Certainly those who are close to us know "how we are," but, again, people are motivated by their own needs and their own fears. People generally focus on themselves and are working on managing their own issues. Other people also want us to understand "how they are." To avoid this expectation that others simple know, it is best to focus on our needs, at any given time, and refrain from expecting others to read our minds. Unexpressed needs and desires are rarely satisfied.

10) **Others should be responsible for my emotional well-being**. Our romantic partners are part of our emotional support system and we are emotionally bonded to them. However, they are not responsible for our well-being. Only we can manage our own emotions and identify our own needs. Being aware of our own needs and fears, communicating clearly, expressing our needs and desires, and managing our own emotions with the tools taught in this book, are key to

creating our own happiness. Believing that you, not others, are responsible for your own happiness and well-being is an excellent place to start. Others may contribute to your happiness, but they cannot make you happy. Only you can do that.

11) **Others should do what I want to do.** We all know someone who has to have everything their way. If you do not know someone like this, it may be you. The problem with this expectation, and the behavior that results, is that others will develop resentment toward you. This resentment ultimately undermines healthy relationships. If this applies to you, consider creating more balance and consciously participating in the activities and choices of others. If you tend to avoid expressing your interests and desires to others, consider speaking up so that others do not always have to make decisions about what to do. This consideration adds balance to relationships and it goes a long way toward eliminating the kinds of situations that lead to resentment.

Complete the following worksheet to begin the work of creating balance in your expectations of yourself and others. In the left-hand column, identify expectations that you encounter in your life. In the middle column, identify an example. In the right-hand column, see if you can make an adjustment in your thinking to create a new (more realistic) expectation.

EXPECTATIONS WORKSHEET

EXPECTATION	EXAMPLE	NEW EXPECTATION
1. Life should be fair.		
2. Opportunities will fall in my lap.		
3. Everyone should like me.		
4. People should agree with me.		
5. People should know what I mean.		
6. I'm going to fail.		
7. I will be happy once I get…		
8. I can change him/her.		
9. Others should know "how I am."		
10. Others should be responsible for my emotional well-being.		
11. Others should do what I want to do.		

HOMEWORK DAY 16

ONE FALSEHOOD SPOILS A THOUSAND TRUTHS. – AFRICAN PROVERB

1) Complete Expectations worksheet.

2) Identify daily gratitude.

3) Conduct exposure therapy and take another break from ABC worksheets.

4) Make a commitment to complete Day 17.

GREAT JOB TODAY! YOU GOT THIS!!!

DAY 17 MAKING GOOD CHOICES

Today's Objective: 1) Learn a simple framework for making choices 2) Explore decision-making in various areas of life

In today's lesson, we will take a hard look at the choices we make and the outcomes they generate. Requiring of yourself that you make good choices substantially improves your overall functioning and optimizes your life outcomes.

Insofar as making decisions is concerned, the following simple formula should become your mantra:

Good Choices = Good Outcomes

Bad Choices = Bad Outcomes

Bad Choices ≠ Good Outcomes

In other words, good choices in life lead to good outcomes. Bad choices in life lead to bad outcomes. You cannot make bad choices in life and expect good outcomes.

This concept applies to every aspect of our lives, including; money, family, marriage, friends, co-workers, alcohol, drugs, careers, everything!

I cannot make poor choices with money and think that I can create financial security. I cannot take my spouse for granted, put very little effort into my marriage, and then wonder why my spouse is unhappy. I cannot have an active addiction and think that there will be no repercussions or consequences for my behavior.

One difficulty in substantiating the legitimacy of this formula is that there is not always an immediate or apparent repercussion for some behaviors. If I drive home drunk one night, there may not be any repercussions. However, this formula inevitably applies to our lives over time. I may never get caught drinking and driving but I may. The more I do, the more I rely on suffering no consequences, the greater the likelihood of them. In this way, not getting caught or experiencing negative consequences may positively reinforce a bad choice. However, over time, making poor choices will eventually lead to poor outcomes. Poor decision making in one area of our lives leads to believing that poor choices in other areas of our lives will work for us in some way, as well.

Consider the following questions in the framework of the formula:

<u>Money</u>

Do I spend less than I make?
Am I irresponsible with money?
Do my money habits negatively affect or impact any relationships in my life? If so, how?
Am I on track to have financial security in my future?
Do I over-save and miss out on enjoying life?

At the end of the day we all must live on a budget and spend less than we make. If I make $75,000, I can't live on a budget of $76,000 or $100,000. Even the Rockefellers cannot spend more than they earn. Whether your budget is small or large, living beyond your means is a house of cards – eventually it falls. Learn to live within your means and you will find a sense of peace that no amount of money can buy.

I highly recommend Dave Ramsey's books or his class, Financial Peace University, for help with finances. Live by his principles, do what he says and you will have financial peace and security. He offers books, classes, DVDs, and various media outlets to help. Start listening to his free podcast. Listening to his podcast will help to create a healthy mindset about money. If your life is out of control and you don't know where to start, start here. Money stressors are a tremendous source of depression and anxiety.

Here are a few basics to know about healthy finances:

Live on a budget. Living on a budget of less than you make is imperative for financial well-being. A monthly budget is comprised of how much money you have coming in and an itemization of every single dollar going out. Your income MUST exceed your expenditures.

When it comes to doing a budget, here are a few suggestions:

- Write it down.

- Savings is crucial. If you cannot save money, you must cut back on lifestyle.

- Yes, you can work more than 40 hours per week. If you need more income, work more – start a side business, sell things from the back of your closet, wait tables – do what you need to do to get your finances in order. We have a culture and mindset of turning wants into needs. Be abnormal and live below your means.

- Question everything. Do I really need cable? Do I really need a new smartphone? Do I really need a land line? Can I spend less on clothes?

- Whatever you have in a car, get a cheaper one. Cars are one of the worst expenditures we make – they go down in value. Minimize what you spend on a car.

- Make savings automatic. If you wait to see what is left over at the end of the month, you will always find something to spend money on. If your savings is first and it is drafted from your account, you will learn to live on the rest.

- When you create your budget, list your items in descending order according to priority. For example, savings, then food and utilities, then shelter, then transportation, then insurance (car, life, health, etc.), then clothing, then you can begin to prioritize lifestyle items. You will be shocked at how you rethink spending money once you begin to pay attention to where your money goes.

- If you have an irregular income, determine what your average income is and use this amount for budgeting purposes. Then, create an 'ups and downs' account. When you have a higher than normal check, put the excess into the account. When you have a lower than normal check, you can draw from the account to bring the amount up to average. For irregular incomes, such as people who work in sales, it is always best to budget less than your average to avoid problems.

- Don't compare your lifestyle to others. You always lose when you compare yourself to others because we always compare ourselves in ways where we fall short. Someone else will always have a nicer house, a nicer car, nicer clothes, and a better vacation.

- Don't use "should" or "I deserve" language when it comes to money. These attitudes rob us of our financial and mental well-being. What we deserve is to educate ourselves about money, make a choice to avoid common habits that most people accept as normal, and create financial security for ourselves.

Relationships

Do I make poor choices in relationships?
Do I have a healthy relationship with my family? With my spouse? With my partner? With my friends? With my coworkers?
Do my relationships need improvement? A little? A lot?
What relationships need improvement?
What needs to be improved with what person?
What can I do to improve these relationships? Time? Effort? Communication? Acceptance?

The nature of all relationships is that there is a dynamic between two individuals that makes for a unique combination based on what each person brings to the relationship. Relationships are fascinating. So often, we focus on the other person – what the other person did, didn't do, said, or didn't say.

When we become self-aware and conscious of ourselves and our effect on others, it is amazing what can happen with the various relationships in our lives. We will address relationships further on Day 27. For now, begin to examine the various relationships in your life, from the closest to the most distant, from the perspective of your contribution. Ask yourself, "What do I contribute to this relationship?" rather than "What do I get from this relationship?"

<u>Substances</u>

Do drugs and/or alcohol have a big or small role in my life?
Why do I drink alcohol? Why do I use drugs?
Do others comment on my use?
Am I known for these behaviors (do I have a reputation)?
Do drugs or alcohol ever create problems for me in my life?
Do I fail to meet any important obligations because of drugs or alcohol?
Can I stop using drugs or alcohol with no difficulty or would it be at all difficult?
Do I spend a significant amount of money on drugs or alcohol?
Does drug or alcohol use impact my relationships in any way?

These questions can be asked of any addiction, from gambling, to sex, to shopping, or to our smartphones. Addiction is complicated but the common threads across all addictions are 1) the compulsive nature of the behavior despite the consequence 2) the avoidance or numbing of unpleasant or painful emotions and 3) the negative impact on some area of our lives.

At the end of the day, not much will improve in our lives as long as there is an active addiction present in our lives. Even though some addictions are more socially acceptable than others (sex, shopping versus heroin), the way to overcome the addiction is the same – face and confront its existence, then tackle the cause of it. Until you resolve the underlying cause, you will never overcome the addiction.

For many, trauma treatment may be necessary. For others, addiction may be a way to self-medicate a serious mental health disorder, such as Bipolar Disorders or Borderline Personality Disorder. There is no need to feel shame about seeking treatment and help for an addiction, as it is all too common in our society. Find a 12-step program or a competent addictions therapist for help in this area of your life.

When you approach these areas of your life – money, relationships, substances, etc. with a healthy attitude and good decision making, watch the changes unfold! As you begin making good choices, your outcomes will improve.

Remember, every bad choice you make is an obstacle you are putting in your own way of achieving a great life.

Use the Good Outcomes Worksheet to analyze your decision-making skills and identify alternative choices. In the first column, identify the area of your life where a decision was made. In the next column, identify the choice you made. A choice is a behavior, not an excuse. Next, see if you can identify why you made the choice you made. Identify the outcome of your choice, then identify another choice you could have made and think about how the outcome would have been different.

GOOD OUTCOMES WORKSHEET

Type of Decision	Poor Choice I Made	Why	Outcome	Alternative Choice	Possible Alternative Outcome
Example: Relationship - Marriage	I cheated on my husband.	I was lonely. I was angry. I wasn't communicating with him. I didn't tell him how I was feeling. I reacted to my impulses and attraction to someone else. I justified my behavior by telling myself he was making me unhappy.	Almost destroyed our marriage and family. The aftermath is worse than the original problem.	Tell him how I felt. Get marriage counseling. Recognize my attraction was a reflection of my frustration in my marriage.	Not cause as much damage to my marriage and family.

HOMEWORK DAY 17

1) Complete the Good Outcomes worksheet.

2) Identify daily gratitude.

3) Conduct exposure therapy and complete an ABC worksheet on any situation.

4) Make a commitment to complete Day 18.

KEEP UP THE GOOD WORK!!!

DAY 18 BEHAVIOR CHANGE

Today's Objective: 1) Identify standards of conduct 2) Increase motivation to improve personal standards of conduct 3) Incorporate standards of conduct into behavioral choices

Most of us don't give much thought to the factors that motivate our behavior or influence our choices. We do what works for us. We make choices based on what was modeled for us and what we were taught as children (which usually coincide). Alternatively, our behavior manifests from an emotional reaction or gut instinct in the moment.

In today's lesson, we will examine the process of putting conscious thought into what motivates the behavioral choices we make. This lesson will also introduce a framework of six standards of conduct toward making more ethical choices. Remember, good choices lead to good outcomes.

The purpose and motivation for today's lesson is to begin to consciously act in a way that is congruent with our core values, which we examined on Day 13. When we act in accordance with strong positive values, we are able to withstand criticism and overcome self-scrutiny. Living in accordance with our values also staves off depression and anxiety.

Behaving in a way that is grounded in ethical standards of conduct will positively affect your well-being and your self-esteem. Good decision-making also builds greater character.

In life, it is what you do, not what you intend, that morally counts. No one sees or cares to understand what your intentions were. All that is seen by others are the outcomes of your behaviors. In other words, if we fail to define ourselves, our behavior will define us. When we take the time to define ourselves in positive ways, that will guide our behavior.

First, let's take a look at the concept of motivation before we introduce the six standards of conduct.

When we consider why people do what they do, it is important to consider the concepts of extrinsic and intrinsic motivation.

Extrinsic motivation is a system whereby a physical reward is exchanged for a specific desired behavior. A classic example is bribing a child with a toy or candy in exchange for "good" behavior. The problem with extrinsic motivation is that, over time, it diminishes the desire for intrinsic motivation, or motivation that is generated internally. Generally, as we grow, our behaviors should become increasingly intrinsically-motivated.

Let's examine the six standards of conduct that govern ethical and prosocial behavior. These standards provide a solid framework that guides and informs good, intrinsically-motivated decisions.

THE SIX STANDARDS OF CONDUCT					
Trustworthiness	Respect	Responsibility	Fairness	Caring	Citizenship

The six standards of conduct include *trustworthiness, respect, responsibility, fairness, caring, and citizenship.* Think about how it feels to be surrounded by people with these traits, and consider incorporating these characteristics into your way of being. Life is easier and more pleasant when we exude and include these standards in our own personal code of conduct.

Think about how these character traits dovetail with boundaries. The lessons in this book are not meant to be mutually exclusive but, rather, are meant to build upon each other. Today's lesson is an important expansion upon the boundaries lesson.

TRUSTWORTHINESS

As we move toward trustworthiness, healthy boundaries will naturally follow. When we conduct ourselves in a trustworthy manner, relationships improve and we will not feel the need to monitor others or to be monitored.

Being able to demonstrate trustworthiness is crucial to healthy, stable relationships. Think about the attachment concepts discussed on Day 15. Human beings are unwilling to attach to others they experience as untrustworthy because an inability to trust another person represents a potential psychological danger – pain!

Trustworthiness involves more than refraining from stealing, lying, cheating, and deception. To further understand trustworthiness, consider the components of being trustworthy: *honesty, integrity, reliability, and loyalty.*

TRUSTWORTHINESS			
Honesty	**Integrity**	**Reliability**	**Loyalty**

Honesty

Possessing the trait of honesty can be expressed in two ways: *honesty in our communications and honesty in our conduct.*

HONESTY	
Honesty in Communications • Truthfulness • Sincerity • Candor	**Honesty in Conduct**

When we are honest in our communications with others, we express ourselves with the purpose of enhancing relationships, not with the purpose of making others see our perspective. However, the obligation to be honest does not give us license to say whatever we are thinking without considering the impact on others.

Three dimensions comprise honesty in communications: *truthfulness, sincerity, and candor.*

Being truthful in communications with others is more than refraining from lying or avoiding lying by omission. Being truthful involves communicating factually, even when it is difficult to do. Being truthful in communication may involve being wrong at times, but being truthful in our correction is important to building and restoring trust. One lie, even a small one, can destroy trust deeply and sometimes permanently.

Being sincere means communicating with a spirit of being genuine. Acts of silence, taking statements out of context, telling partial truths, purposely refraining from clarifying incorrect interpretations are all examples of disingenuousness, which impairs sincerity in communications.

Speaking with candor is often confused with blurting out whatever comes to mind or being inconsiderate of the effect of our words on others. When speaking with candor, one must consider the boundaries of others. Candor includes speaking frankly and sharing information voluntarily that is crucial to facilitating understanding. Remember, honesty without compassion is often just cruelty. When we are candid about topics that are painful to others, we need to be mindful of our delivery.

Honesty in conduct involves behaving in a way that conforms to the rules of society and considers the rights of others. Cheating and stealing violate the rights of others. Cheating and stealing harm relationships and these behaviors also harm us personally by devaluing our moral composition and character.

Integrity

Conducting ourselves with integrity means behaving in accordance with our core values. A person with integrity does not change their values or behaviors depending upon the situation. They do not conform to requests for behaviors that are objectionable to their personal code of conduct, but rather they act from a place of being complete and unified with their values.

A person with integrity is trusted because what you see is what you get. There are no incongruent, deceptive, or nefarious intentions with a person of integrity. People of integrity are predictable and we can rely on their ability to do what is right.

Alternatively, think about how frustrating hypocrites are – they say one thing and do another. Or they have one set of rules for themselves and another set of rules for others. People of integrity avoid these pitfalls.

Reliability

Being reliable means that others can count on us to do what we say we will do, which strengthens relationships. Being reliable means adhering to our moral code to follow through despite any desire to do what is easy or convenient.

Components of being reliable include avoiding insincere excuses, avoiding promises that you cannot or do not want to keep, and avoiding ambiguous commitments.

Loyalty

Loyalty is the commitment of friendship, support, allegiance, dedication, fidelity, and duty toward someone or something. The duty of being loyal extends beyond caring. It creates a sense of importance, value, and respect in others, which strengthens relationships.

Not everyone and every situation warrants your unshakable loyalty. Clearly, there are times when loyalty is not warranted. Loyalty can be complicated.

You have a right to limit your loyalty to the point when your loyalty is no longer in your own best interests and is not appreciated or reciprocated. For example, if you are not appreciated at your job and you have the ability to earn a better living elsewhere, your loyalty is not justified.

You will also have times when your loyalties conflict and you must prioritize them. For example, your loyalty to your children will supersede your loyalty to your job in certain instances. If your child is sick, then that presentation will have to wait!

The most complicated aspect of loyalty is knowing when protecting your own self-interests must supersede loyalty to others.

RESPECT

To fully grasp the concept of respect, consider the Boundaries lesson from Day 2. Respect involves treating yourself and others with consideration; treat others how you would like to be treated.

You can strongly disagree with the behavior of another person but still treat them with respect. All of us should be treated with a baseline amount of respect.

A respectful person treats others with civility, courtesy, and decency. Each individual is considered with dignity, autonomy, tolerance, and acceptance. Acceptance does not include agreement with the behavior or view of someone else, but a recognition that we all have free will and that everyone has inherent worth.

RESPONSIBILITY

Being responsible means being accountable for our own actions and choices. Think about the formula from yesterday's lesson; good choices generate good outcomes.

Holding ourselves accountable, pursuing excellence, and exhibiting self-control all strengthen and fortify our character.

Accountability

Individuals who hold themselves accountable are able to own their mistakes without projecting blame onto others. Those who hold themselves accountable are authentic and take action to make amends. The proper way to make amends will be discussed on Day 20.

Pursuit of Excellence

When we are diligent in our pursuit of excellence, our lives improve when others can rely on our skills. Doing a job that is "good enough" does not challenge us to become the best version of ourselves. Obstacles are seen as barriers to overcome, rather than reasons to stop.

Self-Control

"Children do what feels good. Adults devise a plan and follow it." – Dave Ramsey. The sacrifice of short-term impulses for long-term gain is the hallmark of maturity. Delaying gratification results in better overall well-being, resulting in lower levels of depression and anxiety. A classic example is living on a budget. When we live on a budget and delay impulse purchases, financial security is developed over time.

FAIRNESS

Individuals who exhibit fairness have the ability to exercise what is right without regard to their own feelings or agendas. Similar situations are treated in an equitable, systematic manner.

Having a system in place enables disagreement to be settled in an impartial manner. Consider fairness in the context of the workplace. When fair systems exist, all workers are treated in an equitable manner without regard to emotion or favoritism.

CARING

Caring about the welfare of others is essential for human connection. We cannot expect of others what we ourselves are not willing to give. In other words, we cannot expect others to care about us if we do not care about other people.

Many people think they can make it in this world alone, but humans have an innate need to be connected to others. Even the most introverted among us has a need to connect with other people.

Caring about others fosters the expression of the best part of ourselves and is crucial in the development of empathy.

In today's world of scarcity, caring has taken a backseat to our busy lives and a focus on the self. Caring about others has become an increasingly conscious task.

CITIZENSHIP

Expanding upon caring, citizenship involves caring about our role in a functioning community. Being a good citizen means obeying laws and being a net contributor rather than a net taker. There is a level of responsibility associated with being part of a community that is traded for the benefits and freedoms that come from a being a community member.

Benefits of good citizenship include pride, connection, motivation, inspiration, contacts, and opportunity. Good communities are developed from member contributions and, in turn, the overall lives of community members are enhanced.

A group of individuals gathering to clean up the streets of a downtown area make the community more livable and provide a sense of service and pride to those involved.

On a scale of 1 – 10, rate how closely you are aligned with ethical traits, with 1 being closely and strongly aligned with the trait and 10 representing how far away from the trait you are.

TRAIT	1	2	3	4	5	6	7	8	9	10
TRUSTWORTHINESS										
Honesty										
Honesty in Communications										
Truthfulness										
Sincerity										
Candor										
Honesty in Conduct										
Integrity										
Reliability										
Loyalty										
RESPECT										
RESPONSIBILITY										
Accountability										
Pursuit of Excellence										
Self-Control										
FAIRNESS										
CARING										
CITIZENSHIP										

For any item marked 3 or more, identify the trait in the left-hand column. In the right-hand column, identify one way you can improve your standard of conduct.

Example: Candor	*Use healthy communication skills and express myself more often.*

HOMEWORK DAY 18

1) Complete the Behavior Change rating chart and improvement worksheet.

2) Identify daily gratitude.

3) Conduct exposure therapy and take a break from ABC worksheets.

4) Make a commitment to complete Day 19.

YOU ARE DOING IMPORTANT WORK! KEEP GOING!!!

DAY 19 TEMPERAMENTS

Today's Objective: 1) Learn about temperaments 2) Discover your own temperament 3) Use information about temperaments to further journey of self-discovery

In today's lesson, we will learn about the four temperaments. What is a temperament? A temperament is a grouping of traits that are innate to an individual and contribute to behavior. Our temperament is part of our genetic makeup and contributes to our behavioral tendencies.

While our temperament is inherited and passed on to us as part of our DNA, much like the color of our eyes, our personality is also shaped and influenced by our environments. Our environment, such as our early experiences with our primary caregivers, can suppress or express genetic predispositions.

Consider a baby that is predisposed to being shy but is raised and surrounded by extroverted family members. Outgoing behaviors will be strongly modeled for the child and strongly rewarded when exhibited by the child.

Human personalities are generally categorized into extroverts and introverts. Within each of these two categories are two temperaments, giving us four human temperaments.

EXTROVERT		INTROVERT	
CHOLERIC	SANGUINE	MELANCHOLY	PHLEGMATIC

Extroverts, consisting of the choleric and sanguine temperament types, are more outgoing, more uninhibited in social settings, and generally comfortable around other people. They feel energized in social situations and dislike too much alone time.

Introverts are shy, feel inhibited and anxious in social settings, especially if they are the center of attention. Introverts are comfortable with plenty of alone time instead of socializing.

Let's explore the extroverted temperaments, choleric and sanguine.

Cholerics are outgoing, leaders, and very ambitious. Think of the "Type A" personality. They are driven by success and are goal-oriented. They tend to be controlling, decisive, and sometimes insensitive. In work settings, they perform very well but can overlook the feelings of others. At work, they are self-sufficient, easily admit and correct mistakes, are organized, goal-oriented, production-oriented, visionary, and are good at motivating others. Cholerics do not do well answering to others and prefer being the leader. They easily take charge and are not afraid to make necessary changes.

Cholerics can also struggle in work settings. They can be difficult, bossy, demanding, controlling, irritable, intolerant, and argumentative. Because they demand quality work, from themselves and others, they tend to struggle with relationships and have few friends. Being extroverted, this combination leaves them susceptible to depression and mood swings. However, cholerics are also very passionate, high-energy planners and thrive on mutual respect. Overall, cholerics are strong on the organizational and extroverted dimensions.

Sanguines are people-oriented and talkative. They are expressive and enthusiastic with others. They exude excitement with others and are affectionate. They are described as social, charming, warm, pleasant, creative, compassionate, funny, friendly, and inspirational. Sanguines dislike alone time and become bored when not surrounded by people. Their optimism causes them to be liked by many people and they tend to have many friends.

The carefree nature of sanguines makes them prone to being flighty, disorganized, and having difficulty with completing tasks. They lose track of time easily and may be frequently late and/or forgetful frequently. Overall, sanguines are strong relationally and are described as extroverts.

Now, let's explore the introverted temperaments, melancholy and phlegmatic.

Melancholy temperaments are thinkers. They enjoy having high standards of quality but are less concerned about being right. They are conscientious and are motivated by following the rules. They are detail-oriented, analytical, focused, logical, and deliberate.

Melancholies tend to be deeply affected by traumatic world events and are prone to depression. They are sensitive and easily hurt by others. They need feedback and reassurance from others, and their decision-making style tends to be protracted. They fear making the wrong decision and avoid taking risks. Overall, the melancholy temperament is strong on the organizational dimension.

Phlegmatics are service-oriented and tend to be watchers. They are passive, slow-moving, unemotional, agreeable, patient, indecisive, calm, rational, and considerate. They value family relationships, care about the feelings of others, and forge strong attachments to others. They are good team players and show a sincere, genuine interest in others.

Phlegmatics are not especially ambitious and lack a sense of urgency when completing tasks. They can be loyal to a fault, often having difficulty ending relationships despite the behavior of others. They are resistant to change and prefer consistency. They can experience difficulty with decisions and completing tasks due to their passivity. Overall, they are strong relationally and are introverted.

As you consider which temperament applies to you, reflect on the Childhood Abuse Beliefs Worksheet and the negative beliefs statements. If you tell yourself "I should be more social and outgoing," perhaps a temperament that is more introverted is at play. Part of the purpose of today's lesson of educating yourself about temperaments is self-awareness and self-acceptance. Accepting that your nature is to be more outgoing or more introverted is key to eliminating the inner turmoil of requiring yourself to be someone you are not. We are all unique in the way we relate to others and respond to our life experiences.

Considering which temperament most closely aligns with you, answer the following self-discovery questions:

What is your activity level? Do you tend to be more active or more passive?

What is your natural response to new situations – do you approach or withdraw?

Do you have a tendency to react with a positive mood or a negative mood?

Do you have a tendency to react with intense emotions or calm emotions?

How do you handle situations that require adaptability?

How persistent are you when completing tasks?

HOMEWORK DAY 19

YOU HAVE YOUR WAY. I HAVE MY WAY. AS FOR THE RIGHT WAY, THE CORRECT WAY, AND THE ONLY WAY, IT DOES NOT EXIST.   – FRIEDRICH NIETZSCHE

1) Complete temperament self-discovery questions.

2) Identify daily gratitude.

3) Conduct exposure therapy and complete an ABC worksheet on any situation.

4) Make a commitment to complete Day 20.

YOU GOT THIS!!!

DAY 20 REPAIRING WOUNDS

Today's Objective: 1) Learn how to effectively repair emotional damage 2) Begin to implement changes in the way you make amends and strengthen relationships

Emotional pain is a universal human experience. Sadly, all of us have been hurt deeply by someone we love and trust. In turn, we have also hurt others. In today's lesson, we will explore healthy ways to heal ourselves from scars from emotional pain.

Generally, when we wish to remedy a hurt we caused someone, we apologize and explain our intentions (or lack thereof). For example:

Apology: "I'm so sorry."

Intentions: "I didn't mean to…." "It didn't mean anything." "I wasn't thinking." "It wasn't what you think it was." "I would never hurt you on purpose."

While all of these statements may be true, they do not actually heal the damage caused from lying, betrayal, or cheating.

Keep in mind, apologies are still necessary, appropriate, and desired. However, do not expect them, alone, to heal the hurt because they are not the remedy.

Here is what people need in order to heal:

1) <u>Validation and Empathy</u>

<u>Validation</u>: Acknowledge the person's feelings. Clearly express to the injured person that their feelings make sense and are valid. Do not minimize. Don't add "but" to the end of any sentence. Tell the person that what they feel is real. Do not try to veto the hurt by pointing out how you have been hurt by things the wounded person has done, even when it involves the same behavior. Keep the conversation focused on the injured person, and avoid shifting the conversation focus to yourself.

<u>Empathy</u>: Empathy is defined as the ability to understand and share the feelings of another. In other words, "When you feel something, I feel something. I hurt because you hurt." The person who has been hurt will have difficulty healing when they carry the pain and burden of the offense. Empathy is key to reestablishing a balance in the relationship. Validating and sharing in their pain helps bridge the gap created by the injury.

When we are hurt and in pain, it is difficult to heal when we are alone in our pain. For example, in the case of cheating in relationships, couples often hesitate to address the issue past the initial discussions for fear of making it worse, especially during calm and pleasant times. When things seem to be returning to "normal", it is understandable to be inclined to "let sleeping dogs lie," but the person who has been wounded often perceives this dynamic as a free pass to escape experiencing the consequences of their choice. This scenario unwittingly plants the seeds of resentment.

2) Assurances that it won't happen again

People will not fully recover and choose to psychologically reattach to someone they perceive to be a psychological threat. If you have deeply wounded me and I believe there is any chance that will happen again, I cannot trust you at that level. Until trust is restored, the relationship cannot be repaired.

There are several ways to create assurances; each relationship and circumstance may require different approaches. Some forms of assurances include demonstrating insight, being an open book, changing behaviors, initiating conversations, and making sacrifices.

Insight is a key component to assurances that the hurt will not be repeated. If the person inflicting the pain does not know why they did what they did, then that lack of insight does not provide the wounded party sufficient reassurance that the event will not recur. For example, if a spouse cheats and blames the circumstances, rather than recognizing his/her need for excitement and external validation and accepting responsibility, then healing will not occur. The behavior can be forgiven, but forgiveness is different than healing.

Being an open book is important to reestablishing trustworthiness. A person who has nothing to hide should hide nothing, including such behaviors as being accountable for time and money, as well as social media and cell phones. Removing passcodes and offering passwords to email and social media is a demonstration of trustworthiness. That being said, checking on a partner, especially habitual and obsessive checking, does not provide assurances. It is the gesture and concept of being open that reestablishes trust, not the process of seeking and not finding. The reassurance is in the gesture – not the investigation.

Any behaviors associated with hurting others bear changing. For example, if a partner or spouse has a gambling problem that he/she was hiding, the behavior of going to the casino must change. If spending time away from home led to an affair, then that behavior must change. If behaviors stay the same, it does not demonstrate any willingness to make sacrifices for the relationship. Significantly, it also does not provide the necessary assurances that the event/offenses won't recur.

The wounded individual should not have the burden of initiating conversations about the healing process. The party who perpetrated the pain should undertake the active role of having conversations and check-ins with the injured party. This gesture shows a willingness to heal the relationship and demonstrates a level of caring concern about the harm inflicted. These conversations are difficult and humbling because they require that the perpetrator face his/her own mistakes and feel the associated shame for what he/she has done.

Making sacrifices for the benefit of the injured party and the relationship is one of the most powerful and important tools for healing relationships. Making sacrifices sends the message that you are vested in the relationship; and the relationship is important enough to make a sacrifice.

For example, if an affair occurred at work, a partner may change jobs. If an affair happened with someone locally, the couple may move to a new area. These extreme sacrifices send a crucial message that the relationship is worth making big changes to preserve and protect it.

The 95-5 Rule

A general rule of thumb for the healing process is that the person who perpetrated the hurt is 95% responsible for repairing the damage that they caused. It is not the responsibility of the wounded partner to "get over it," nor should they be told that the burden is theirs to trust again as in "you just need to learn to trust me again." The perpetrator is the one who must earn and establish trust, as they are the one who broke it. That being said, the wounded partner must not remain in the victim role and is responsible for accepting overtures at healing and repairing of the relationship. It takes both parties to heal and recover but the bulk of the burden should always be placed with the person who caused the damage.

Practice a new way of making amends by apologizing with validation, empathy, and offering assurances that it won't happen again. Use a current example or make new amends with an example from the past. Consider a spouse, a partner, a friend, a family member, or a co-worker. Answer the questions below to assess how well you did.

What was the situation for which you made amends?

With whom did you make amends?

How did you validate? What emotions were recognized?

How did you empathize? What did you say?

What was the response to the validation and empathy from the other person?

What assurances did you offer?

What was the response to the assurances from the other person?

How do you feel about making the amends?

HOMEWORK DAY 20

1) Complete repairing wounds exercise and questions.

2) Identify daily gratitude.

3) Conduct exposure therapy and take a break from ABC worksheets.

4) Make a commitment to complete Day 21.

GREAT WORK TODAY!!!

DAY 21 REACTIVE VERSUS RESPONSIVE

Today's Objective: 1) Learn how to further control emotional and behavioral reactions 2) Identify vulnerabilities 3) Learn the STOP strategy to become more responsive

Today's lesson dovetails with Day 1, ABC Worksheets. Hopefully, you have been practicing the worksheets with your daily homework in order to fully integrate the cognitive process. Remember when we talked about the cognitive process, we learned to identify emotions and thought distortions, then reframe them to create healthier thinking and emotions.

But, what happens when your emotions are so intense that you become *reactive*? What happens when you are overwhelmed? What happens when you have difficulty stopping your reactive behaviors?

Speaking of stopping, we will learn a strategy using the acronym STOP. Practicing STOP, in conjunction with the ABC process, will help you learn to become less *reactive* and, in turn, more *responsive*.

The concept of becoming more responsive and less reactive is part of Dialectical Behavior Therapy, which is indicated for many mental health disorders, particularly Borderline Personality Disorder. Individuals diagnosed with Borderline Personality Disorder tend to experience difficulty managing emotional reactions.

So what causes people to be so emotionally reactive? As you now know, it is not the situation that causes emotional reactivity, it is our thought process that generates our emotions that lead to our behavioral responses.

For those individuals with underlying vulnerabilities, such as trauma and neglect, triggering events can easily result in reactivity.

Think about a person who has just lost a pet. Watching an SPCA commercial is going to be a triggering event for a person who has an underlying vulnerability of grief from a recent loss, which will generate an emotional reaction of sadness (and probably a physiological response of crying).

Becoming fully aware of your own personal vulnerabilities can be a powerful exercise in preparing your mental health toolbox. When you are aware of your own vulnerabilities, it will enable you to become less reactive because you will no longer be blind-sided by triggering events.

Take a moment to explore your own vulnerabilities after reviewing the following example. First, identify what types of situations cause the most distress for you? Next, identify the emotions you tend to feel. Lastly, see if you can identify the root cause of these vulnerabilities.

VULNERABILITY		SOURCE
SITUATION/TRIGGER	**EMOTIONS**	
Examples: Dating – being hurt in a relationship.	Abandoned Unloved Worthless	Emotional abuse and neglect from my mother.
People leaving – ending encounters with others.	Abandoned Disliked	Emotional abuse and neglect from my mother.
Misbehaving kids.	Disrespected Abandoned Unloved	Emotional abuse and neglect from my mother. Low self-esteem.
Someone calling me out for being a know-it-all.	Humiliated	Being berated and humiliated as a child by my mother.

Owning your own vulnerabilities is a key component of moving toward being responsive, rather than being reactive. It also allows you to fully grasp the concept that nothing is personal – everyone has vulnerabilities!

Using the acronym of STOP will further assist with the process of becoming more responsive.

S	Stop	Focus on stopping yourself. Do not react.
T	Take a breath	Don't worry if anyone thinks you are strange. Inhale and exhale at least once, ten times if you need to!
O	Observe	Notice what you are saying to yourself and how you are interpreting the situation. Put words to what you are feeling. If possible, see if you can identify any vulnerabilities. Ask yourself: Am I being realistic? Am I taking this personally?
P	Plan with perspective	Look at the situation from a broader perspective – what is the bigger picture? Ask what your various options are. We usually get stuck in our automatic reactions and don't consider other alternatives. Think about what you learned on Day 18, Behavior Change, and the values you want to live by.

Now, let's take a look at your typical reactive behaviors and look for ways to become more responsive.

REACTIVE	RESPONSIVE
Examples: Yell at my kids.	Use STOP, address the unwanted behavior, use consequence parenting skills (Day 28), think about parenting on purpose and focus on teaching them rather than punishing them.
Emotionally shutting down, internalizing pain.	Identify emotions, use cognitive skills, use healthy communication skills.
Shutting myself off from people.	Identify emotions, use cognitive skills, use healthy communication skills.
Arguing with my spouse.	Identify emotions, use cognitive skills, use healthy communication skills.

HOMEWORK DAY 21

1) Complete Vulnerabilities worksheet. Complete Reactive versus Responsive worksheet.

2) Identify daily gratitude.

3) Conduct exposure therapy and take a break from ABC worksheets.

4) Make a commitment to complete Day 22.

KEEP IT GOING! YOU'RE DOING GREAT WORK!!!

DAY 22 STRENGTHS AND WEAKNESSES

Today's Objective: 1) Learn the importance of integrating all aspects of yourself 2) Identify strengths and weaknesses 3) Identify areas marked for improvement

Today's lesson expands upon Day 14, Positive Qualities, where the process of identifying and accepting your own special, unique traits began.

The process of developing a positive, healthy self-esteem is one that takes practice using effective tools. Another tool for your mental health tool belt is viewing particular aspects of yourself from a more complex perspective.

Ordinarily, traits and qualities are viewed dichotomously – they are either good or bad.

In today's lesson, we will look at our traits and qualities and work on accepting and integrating them. As you move toward becoming whole, you will begin to feel more content, confident, and at peace.

Think about one of the qualities identified on Day 14. As you consider a quality, remember that you most likely do not exhibit that quality all of the time and it may not be positive, depending on the situation. Even positive qualities may not work to our advantage at all times.

For example, think about having a quality of having strong opinions. This quality may be problematic at times, but useful, or even necessary, at other times.

Begin to think of weaknesses not as negatives, but as attributes that do not come easily to you and as opportunities for improvement.

Remember, it is not possible for all aspects of our personality to be positive. Embrace all of your qualities with a goal of seeking to improve upon yourself. Imagine if you had nothing to work on! Working on yourself is part of the growing process of life. And when we stop growing, we stop living.

Understanding your strengths and weaknesses enables you to maximize your potential, helps you recognize your limitations, focus on your abilities, and improves your self-esteem.

Begin by identifying and creating context for your attributes:

I MAY BE (SOMETHING YOU NEED TO IMPROVE)……..	BUT (POSITIVE ASPECT OF YOU)
Example: I may be too independent	*but I have conquered by fear of being alone*

Now, let's look at where your talents are best used:

I FEEL STRONG/ENERGIZED WHEN I…..	I FEEL WEAK/DRAINED WHEN I…..
Example: I feel energized when I am organizing and cleaning something.	*I feel drained when I have to attend a function where I need to make small talk.*

Every human being has weaknesses, shortcomings, and flaws. Use the following worksheet to identify and begin to accept the parts of yourself that are not ideal. In the first column, identify a weakness, a shortcoming, or a flaw. In the second column, identify what you would tell someone you love who exhibited the same trait. Finally, begin to speak to yourself in this way.

My Weakness, Shortcoming, Flaw	If someone you loved had this trait, what would you say to him or her?
Example: Independent	*There are times when being independent is a good trait. It is okay to ask for help. Asking for help does not make you weak or needy.*

HOMEWORK DAY 22

1) Complete the three strengths and weaknesses exercises.

2) Identify daily gratitude.

3) Conduct exposure therapy and complete an ABC worksheet on any situation.

4) Make a commitment to complete Day 23.

GOOD JOB TODAY! YOU GOT THIS!!!

DAY 23 REFRAME LOSS TO GAIN

Today's Objective: Learn to identify lessons from painful past experiences

Today's lesson is simple but important. When you hear the word "loss," you may think of the passing of someone you love or care about.

But loss can occur in hidden ways in our lives. Loss occurs when you have to say goodbye to something or someone and this evokes sadness. Divorce, retirement, infertility, sending a child off to college, surviving childhood abuse, job change, moving, the death of a pet, can all spur feelings of loss.

We will all experience life events that can generate feelings of loss. It is impossible to pass through this life without painful events.

Reframing the way we interpret these events is key to shifting from suffering to appreciation and gratitude.

Painful events can startle us into an entirely new awareness and help us to become mindfully present and aware of all the wonderful things that surround us.

Losing loved ones is very painful, especially when it is unexpected and tragic. The death of an elderly grandparent can be very sad but is usually easier to process than the tragic loss of a young person. Neither loss is easy; both are accompanied by pain. However, it is generally easier to move past an event that makes sense to us.

Coping with loss involves several important components. First, loss of any kind takes time to process. Your time frame for managing loss is your own. One person's time frame may look very different from another person's time frame.

Allow yourself time to process the loss and to grieve.

Grief from losses can come in waves; it is not a linear process. There may be times when you are feeling better, followed by times that are more difficult. There may be triggering events, such as other losses, or the sadness may pop up or creep in.

An important method for managing losses involves viewing the loss from the perspective of what was gained from the event. In the time closest to the event, it may be very difficult to think about what was gained from the experience. As time passes, it will become easier to search for gratitude.

Review the examples below and complete the Loss/Gain worksheet.

LOSS	GAIN
Example: Got divorced	*I experienced an important journey for myself that would not have happened had I stayed married. I learned independence that I needed, learned about the impact of my childhood abuse on my marriage. I learned to overcome my fear of being alone. I started a new career that would not have occurred if I had stayed married. I have had some great adventures that would not have happened if I had stayed married.*
Betrayed at my job, forced to quit	*I found a better job, make more money, and learned a lesson about limiting my loyalty to an employer. If I had not had a bad experience with my former employer, I would not have had the opportunities I have had with my current employer.*
My father died	*I learned to appreciate those close to me. I make an effort to stay in contact with family members and don't take for granted that they will always be there. Losing a parent has made me more empathetic toward people experiencing grief. I am grateful that he passed quickly and did not suffer for an extended period of time. I am glad I was able to be with him when he was passing away.*
Dog passed away	*I rescued my dog from the pound and gave her a good life. She experienced a lot of love from our family.*
Filed bankruptcy and lost my home	*I was forced to learn how to manage my finances and forced to learn the root of my overspending. My mental health improved due to the experience and learned ways to manage my depression from my childhood abuse. I used to take my home for granted; now I appreciate having a safe roof over my head.*
Neglected and abused as a child	*I used the experience of childhood neglect and abuse to teach myself how to meet my own needs. I work with neglected and abused children and am able to empathize with their experiences and connect with them. My one experience allows me to help hundreds and hundreds of children.*
Retired	*I have the time to spend exploring my creative side. I have time to travel and explore the world. I have the ability to spend my days as I choose and volunteer with causes that are important to me.*
Took my last child to college	*I am able to give her an experience I never had. I did a good job raising my children – they are good people. I have the time to explore my creative side and spend more time with friends.*

LOSS	GAIN

HOMEWORK DAY 23

1) Complete Loss and Gain worksheet.

2) Identify daily gratitude.

3) Conduct exposure therapy and take a break from ABC worksheets.

4) Make a commitment to complete Day 24.

THE FINISH LINE IS IN SIGHT!!!

DAY 24 GOAL SETTING

Today's Objective: 1) Learn the purpose of goal-setting 2) Learn effective methods for setting and achieving goals

Setting goals is a bit of a cliché in today's culture. A standard interview question is "What are your 5 and 10 year goals?" Calendars and planners are making a comeback with many brands and choices available.

One of the reasons that goal-setting is such a common topic is that it is important. You are exponentially more likely to achieve a goal if it is identified and if it is written down.

Living life without goals is like driving around in your car hoping you reach a destination. How will you know if you arrived if you haven't identified the destination? How do you determine the best route to your destination without planning?

Setting goals will move you away from autopilot to a more purposeful movement. Developing an action plan will maximize your efforts, much like creating a route to a destination makes your movements more efficient.

Creating goals will allow you to hold yourself accountable. Many people fear setting goals because of their own fear of failure. Failure is a teacher; failure teaches us what not to do. Failure is not the absence of success; it is the guide toward prosperity. Living well involves learning and failure is merely the opportunity to do so.

Goals create motivation. Those who struggle with motivation tend to lack specific life goals. Motivation enables movement past obstacles, which are inevitable.

For today's lesson, we will explore setting and achieving short-term and long-term goals.

For short-term goals, such as going to the gym X times per week, we must first explore procrastination. They key to overcoming procrastination is two-fold. First, identify negative emotions when thinking about the task to be completed and focus on the positive emotion that will arise when the task is completed. Second, set yourself up for a reward when the task is completed. For example, allow yourself to watch television once the bathroom is cleaned.

Use the following goal worksheet to identify and increase achievement of short-term goals.

Goal/Activity	Goal	Mon	Tues	Weds	Thur	Fri	Sat	Sun	TOTAL

On a scale of 1 to 10, how happy were you this week and why?

| |
| |
| |

What were your 3 greatest achievements this week?

| |
| |
| |

Review your goals and assess your progress. Did you spend your time on the right things? If not, how will you improve next week?

| |
| |
| |

When considering your long-term goals, first consider what areas of your life require your attention. Here are some suggestions:

Family Relationships
Friendships
Social Life
Romantic Relationships
Mental Health
Nutrition/Diet
Physical Health/Exercise
Education
Work/Career
Finances
Retirement
Home/Living Environment
Daily Habits/Self-Care
Spirituality
Actualization/Self-Discovery/Individual Growth
Character/Integrity/Ethics/Values
Purpose
Fun
Community

Long-term goals can be overwhelming, causing paralysis. When considering a long-term goal, break the goal into smaller goals. For example, I may have a goal of opening a business. Opening a business involves many steps, including: selecting an idea, researching it, writing a business plan, finding investors, opening bank accounts, obtaining insurance, filing legal documents, ordering inventory, renting space, hiring employees, etc. All of the steps must be identified and sub-steps for various categories may need to be identified. Each step requires action. Without action, you won't achieve anything.

Set a time frame for achieving long-term goals. Time frames will increase motivation and can be changed, depending upon obstacles. Many people hesitate to make goals and identify time frames because they fear missing the target. Goals and time frames can be flexible and can be revised.

Use the following goal worksheet to identify at least one long-term goal and begin the process of considering short-term goals in the direction of your long-term goal.

Goal:
1.
a.
b.
c.
d.
2.
a.
1.
2.
3.
b.
c.
3.
a.
b.
4.
a.
b.
c.
d.

HOMEWORK DAY 24

1) Complete the weekly goal worksheet and the long-term goal worksheet.

2) Identify daily gratitude.

3) Conduct exposure therapy and complete an ABC worksheet on any situation.

4) Make a commitment to complete Day 25.

KEEP UP THE GREAT WORK! YOU GOT THIS!!!

DAY 25 NARRATIVE THERAPY

Today's Objective: 1) Learn about the rationale for narrative therapy 2) Begin the process of self-acceptance through writing and owning your own story

In today's lesson, narrative therapy will be explored. The concept is actually quite simple. Narrative therapy allows us to compile, explore, question, and incorporate the story of an individual.

Remember in earlier lessons what was learned about how we destructively incorporate painful life experiences into our psyche. Children frequently develop unhealthy belief systems as the result of abuse, neglect, and maltreatment.

Painful experiences are often avoided and positive experiences are minimized. Much suffering comes from the coping skill of emotional numbing.

Owning your own story can be an extremely empowering step on the journey of healing and creating good mental health. It is certainly not possible to go back in time and change our past experiences. Therefore, our only options are 1) to deny or avoid our story or 2) to own and accept our story.

Now that you are becoming more practiced at ABC worksheets, conducting today's exercise will be less frightening than it would have been before your progress utilizing this book. Part of exploring past experiences will involve challenging your prior thoughts about those events, which were probably subconscious and unhealthy, as well as confronting painful emotions.

As you conduct today's exercise, be sure to increase your awareness of your prior and current interpretations, especially if they are childhood experiences and contemporaneous interpretations. Think about the messages you received, directly and indirectly, surrounding these events. Think about how your child brain may have misinterpreted what happened and how it affected you. Also, consider how the adults who surrounded you in childhood shaped your reality.

One of the outcomes of today's lesson is to create a more cohesive sense of self. As an individual evolves into the process of comfortably exploring their experiences, as they process unhealthy thoughts and emotions about those experiences, and as they develop a perspective that fully integrates their experiences, the process of acceptance will begin to unfold. With that acceptance comes healing.

Many people describe themselves as broken. Today's lesson is a reminder that we can heal, and those with scars are often the most interesting, wise, and charismatic among us. We can, with work, be shaped by our experiences without remaining broken by the events.

For today's exercise, you will need a blank wall and a lot of sticky notes. Alternatively, you can use the floor and pieces of paper.

On each note, write down an experience from your life that you remember. The memory can be good, bad, or indifferent. If you remember it, it probably has some meaning to you. As you write down a memory, arrange it on the wall chronologically and horizontally. You can also arrange some of the notes vertically for similar time frames. For example, if you have several memories from kindergarten, you can arrange those vertically. Most people do not remember the exact date of life events.

The exercise should take a while and you may want to work on the exercise over time. As the exercise gets underway, forgotten memories will probably get triggered. If you become emotional, allow yourself to feel your emotions and take a break if needed. You may also need to use ABC worksheets to process some events.

HOMEWORK DAY 25

QUOTE OF THE DAY:

TO LIVE IS TO SUFFER. TO SURVIVE IS TO FIND SOME MEANING IN THE SUFFERING. – FRIEDRICH NIETZSCHE

1) Complete the narrative therapy exercise.

2) Identify daily gratitude.

3) Conduct exposure therapy and take a break from ABC worksheets.

4) Make a commitment to complete Day 26.

ALMOST THERE! YOU GOT THIS!!!

DAY 26 IDENTITY AND PURPOSE

Today's Objective: 1) Learn about concepts of identity, sense of self, and purpose 2) Identify ways we avoid our authentic selves and why 3) Gather more concrete sense of self, individual identity, and purpose

Today's lesson expands upon several previous lessons. Having a solid sense of your own identity is foundational for functioning in all areas of your life. Without a solid sense of self and sense of your purpose, individuals are prone to various difficulties, poor decision-making, addictions, depression, anxiety, and dysfunctional relationships – to name a few.

Individuals without a strong sense of self and purpose report feeling 'lost' and are vulnerable to seeking a sense of self through others, often referred to as codependency. Lacking a strong identity and purpose can lead individuals to put the needs, wants, and emotions of others before their own, which fuels unhappiness.

Identity is the collection of attributes that defines how we see ourselves. When the attributes of our identity are externalized, those attributes control us. Our self of self-worth becomes dependent upon external considerations. True freedom arises when we are not dependent upon something outside of ourselves for the way we feel about ourselves. The way we feel about ourselves begins with the relationship we have with ourselves.

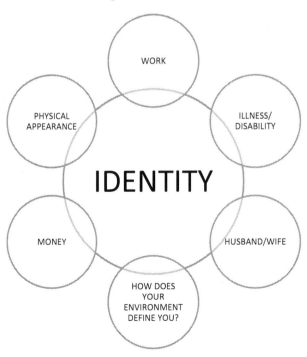

Consider the Identity diagram. Individuals frequently define themselves via external factors, such as work and money. Many people define themselves by what they do for a living. But what if you career ends, or changes? You are still the same person. What if you get divorced and you are no longer a husband? You are still the same person. What if your financial situation changes, or your physical appearance changes drastically? You are still the same person. And yet, many individuals unknowingly define themselves in these ways.

It today's lesson, you will learn to move past these changing, external ways of defining yourself.

To begin to discover your identity, begin by looking at what qualities, traits, characteristics, and values you admire in others. In the following exercise, identify three individuals you admire. These individuals do not need to be people you know. They may be celebrities or historical figures. Identify why you admire them.

1.
    a.

    b.

    c.

    d.

2.
    a.

    b.

    c.

    d.

3.
    a.

    b.

    c.

    d.

Look at your list. Did you list attributes and characteristics, or did you list external qualities? What we tend to admire in others are attributes that we value and often possess ourselves. Looking at what we admire in others is a starting point to discovering our core identity.

Next, we will investigate the obstacles that have gotten in the way of discovering our true selves. Childhood abuse and neglect often contribute to our inability to know who we are. In order to survive our unfavorable experiences, defense mechanisms and masks are born as self-protective measures. These measures prevent the healthy development of identity because the individual is always in self-protection mode, even after leaving the abusive environment. Patterns begin for one reason and continue as automatic responses. Most behavior is adaptive, at the time, but often becomes maladaptive over time.

Let's discover which masks you employ in your life. In the following chart, identify which masks you use for self-protection, determine their origin, when they surface in your life, and then identify one way you can begin to release your reliance upon the mask.

MASK	ORIGIN	CURRENT PRESENCE	LIFE WITHOUT THE MASK
Perfectionist			
Volunteer			
Smart/ Know It All			
Intellectual			
Competent			
Positive/ The Nice Person			
The Loner/ Independent/ I Don't Need Anyone			
Victim/ Dependent			
Tough Guy/ Tough Girl			
Grump			
Fashionista			
The Topper			
Pleaser			
Innocent and Sweet			
Life of the Party			
Comedian			
Wallflower			
Hippie/ Tree Hugger/ Free Love			

Answer the following questions to further explore your core identity:

Who am I?

What makes me special?

Is there a pattern to my life?

Where am I going?

What is my gift?

What is my message?

What is important to me when it comes to how to treat other people?

How do I view money?

Am I creative? Musical? Artistic?

What's missing in my life?

What am I doing when I lose track of time?

What did I want to be as a child?

How do I have fun?

How much importance do I place on family?

How do I approach my fears?

What are my dreams?

If I could do/be anything without limitations, what would I do/be?

Am I positive/negative?

What are my views on the afterlife?

Does everything happen for a reason?

What can I do to contribute to my community/the world?

What are my talents?

What are my hobbies?

What am I proud of?

Do I care what others think of me?

What do others compliment me on?

Who has had the greatest impact on my life? Why?

What do I like to read?

Do I stand up for myself?

Do I listen to my heart?

Do I complete tasks promptly?

What is on my bucket list?

Do I donate to charity?

Do I settle for mediocrity?

Do I forgive myself?

Do I take time for myself?

Am I inquisitive?

If I signed up for a class today, what would the class be?

What are my values?

What are my morals?

Next, let's explore the concept of purpose. Living a life *of* purpose, *on* purpose is the key to satisfaction, peace, and fulfillment. Purpose is a process and not a destination. Our purpose evolves as our lives progress.

The experiences of our lives are often preparation for the fulfillment of our purpose. For example, a child who is victimized in childhood may become a lawyer, fighting for those who have been victimized. Or that same individual may volunteer as a Court Appointed Special Advocate or guardian ad litem (individuals who speak on behalf of children in legal proceedings). Fulfilling your purpose may not involve a career. A child who experienced neglect may find purpose in being a stay-at-home mother and creating a strong, healthy family.

Consider the following questions to begin to uncover your purpose:

What gives me energy?

What excites me?

What kind of ideas come to me in the shower?

What kind of things do people always ask me about?

What kind of advice do others seek from you?

What kind of conversations do I have with those closest to me?

What subject matter do you immerse yourself in with loved ones?

What information do you share with the people you care about most?

What do you talk about when you're being your true self?

What do I do with my free time?

What topics do I regularly read about?

What do I research on the internet when I am bored?

What recurring dreams do I have?

During which experiences in my life have I felt the most alive?

What unique interests, or abilities, did I have as a young child?

What would I be doing if money were no object?

What would I be doing if I absolutely, 100%, did not care about what other people think?

What is on my bucket list?

What topics can I blend together to create my own unique niche?

If I were to write a short (1-2 sentence) *"About Me"*, describing the ideal version of myself, what would it be?

Finally, complete the following exercise to uncover your purpose:

Consider the following question "What is my true purpose in life?" and write the first answer

that pops into your head. It does not need to be a complete sentence; a short phrase or word is

fine.

Next, answer repeatedly until you write the answer that moves you, inspires you, makes you cry,

or makes you want to take action. This answer is your purpose.

HOMEWORK DAY 26

QUOTE OF THE DAY:

*INSTEAD OF SAYING, I'M DAMAGED, I'M BROKEN, SAY I'M HEALING,
I'M REDISCOVERING MYSELF, I'M STARTING OVER. – HORACIO
JONES*

1) Complete the Identity, Masks, and Purpose exercises.

2) Identify daily gratitude.

3) Conduct exposure therapy and complete an ABC worksheet on any situation.

4) Make a commitment to complete Day 27.

YOU'VE GOT THIS!!!

DAY 27 INTIMATE RELATIONSHIPS

Today's Objective: 1) Learn about the nature of intimate relationships 2) Learn what elements are crucial to the healthy functioning of relationships 3) Learn the common areas of relationship dysfunction 4) Learn why typical counseling techniques are ineffective 5) Learn about the different types of abuse 6) Learn the real reasons for cheating 7) Learn the crucial first steps to healing relationships

At some point, most people struggle in intimate relationships. It is frustrating to be in a distressed relationship when you do not know what damaged it or how to fix it. To be a healthy partner, it is important to understand the nature of relationships. Often times, couples argue over trivial matters as opposed to the central issues, which threaten the relationship. This dynamic is why looking beyond your partner's surface complaint is crucial to moving in the direction of healing the relationship.

In today's lesson, we will explore various aspects of relationships that impair healthy relationship functioning, examine some important skills to strengthen the relationship, and use an exercise as a first step in moving both partners in the right direction.

The Nature of Relationships

The essence of adult intimate relationships is that they involve emotional bonds, mirroring the parent-child bond but with a sexual component, that fulfills our biological need for love and belonging. We enter into relationships for companionship wherein we get our emotional, physical, spiritual, and safety needs met.

The reason we are attracted to particular people extends beyond physical attraction and pheromones. There is a reason why we choose certain partners that is important to understand because it relates to relationship discord.

We all come to relationships wounded in some way, often from childhood. Abuse, like all forms of human behavior, occurs on a continuum, from mild to severe. For example, mom behaving in an embarrassing way on the first day of school on one end, to experiences of emotional neglect and physical or sexual abuse on the other end. We are subconsciously drawn to partners who exhibit traits and qualities that mirror those we experienced with our primary caregivers in childhood. As we form an attachment with an intimate partner, those wounds surface in the relationship when our partners exhibit those hurtful traits from our past.

We tend to select and marry our unresolved parent. In that way, we replay painfully disappointing relationship experiences seeking a different outcome. In other words, we seek to resolve that which is unresolved. For example, an individual who grew up with a selfish mother likely felt neglected, unimportant, unloved, and unheard in childhood. That individual is predisposed to selecting selfish partners in an effort to reconcile past wounds. As selfishness appears in the partner, the same emotions from childhood will resurface in an exponentially profound manner, and conflict will arise.

Although relationships between two people are unique, all intimate relationships follow a predetermined set of phases. The first phase is the romantic phase, also known as limerence. In this early phase of a relationship, the two partners are getting to know each other and their brains are flooded with feel-good, bonding chemicals that cause them to begin the attachment process.

Next is the attachment or commitment phase. This phase involves making the decision to remain in the relationship and commit to meeting each other's needs. During the commitment phase, arguments often ensue as emotional vulnerabilities are triggered. Conflict arises when the unspoken expectation of having our needs satisfied falls short of our experience.

Next is the power struggle phase. In this phase, arguments, manipulation, and coercion abound as the partners experience attachment panic and partners attempt to reestablish emotional connectivity with each other. Lacking the ability to move beyond this phase, many couples remain entrenched in the power struggle for long periods of time or until the ultimate demise of the relationship. At the end of today's lesson, guidance will be provided that helps direct couples beyond the struggle and toward success.

Healthy Relationships

Healthy relationships demonstrate several elements, and the following list is a road map to the destination of a mutually satisfying and rewarding relationship.

First, a healthy relationship provides each partner with emotional support, where each person is able to experience protection and safety during times of distress. The relationship provides comfort and solace when partners are able to connect with each other.

Next, partners in healthy relationships feel loved and accepted by one another, even during times of disagreement. Feeling fully accepted, shortcomings and flaws included, is imperative in a nurturing relationship.

In healthy relationships, partners value and appreciate the relationship. The relationship is a priority and time is devoted to nurturing and strengthening it.

Solid relationships are a stable base from which partners explore and experience the world. Each person feels safe in their ability to pursue goals and interests outside of the relationship. These pursuits do not interfere with/result in neglect of the relationship.

A healthy relationship is comprised of two trusting partners. Trust is not limited to faith in a partner's monogamy, but it also encompasses the belief that each partner can rely on the stability of the relationship and that their individual needs will be met.

Intimacy is present in a successful relationship, whereby both partners feel comfortable being vulnerable with each other and freely share their most intimate thoughts and feelings. Healthy boundaries, marked by a balance of dependence and independence, are present in relationships with deep intimacy.

Each individual in a respectful relationship has a strong sense of self-worth that is not dependent upon the relationship. However, each partner contributes to the self-worth of the other partner and does not feel the need to choose between the relationship and their individuality.

Lastly, each partner is able to manage disagreements in an effective, caring manner whereby conflict does not devolve into threats or name-calling. Disagreements do not threaten the relationship, problems are addressed openly, and each partner is able to move on from the conflict.

These elements are goals for a healthy, enduring, and rewarding relationship. For those in a relationship, use the following chart to rate the strength of each element of your relationship (from your perspective) on a scale from 1 (weakest) to 10 (strongest). Consult with your partner and add your partner's scores to the column provided for their assigned rating. Identify weak areas or areas where you see a large discrepancy and mark those in the "Areas to Work On" column.

ELEMENT	RATE FROM 1 TO 10 (ME)	MY PARTNER'S RATING	AREAS TO WORK ON
EMOTIONAL SUPPORT			
FEEL ACCEPTED AND LOVED			
APPRECIATE THE RELATIONSHIP			
SECURE BASE			
TRUST			
COMFORTABLE WITH INTIMACY			
INDIVIDUAL SELF-WORTH			
EFFECTIVE AND CARING MANAGEMENT OF CONFLICTS			

Categories of Relationship Discord

Those who experience the pain of having relationship difficulty often feel alone, ashamed, and think that their problems are unique and cannot be solved. However, there are generally several common categories of relationship discord that surface. These categories include lack of passion, arguing, infidelity, emotional neglect, money stressors, separate lives, lack of affection, lack of sexual satisfaction, lack of trust, and addiction.

Countless couples experience problems in more than one category. Many experience problems in several categories, even all categories, yet stay together. Many people wonder why they cannot leave the relationship, or look at other couples and wonder why they are still together. Two dynamics must be present in order to end a relationship – 1) the cost of being in the relationship must exceed the benefits, and 2) one person must lose hope that the relationship will improve.

Many couples turn to marriage/couples counseling for help.

Counseling

People generally wait until their relationship is on the verge of ending before they seek help. Early intervention before unhealthy patterns become engrained is crucial to salvaging a relationship before irreparable harm is done.

Relationship difficulty usually results from attachment panic. Most approaches to couples counseling focus on developing problem-solving skills, communication skills, and conflict-resolution skills. Unfortunately, teaching these skills only addresses the surface symptoms and this counseling focus ignores the true source of distress.

Couples who are struggling in relationships are experiencing emotional disconnection. The source of their emotional nourishment is fractured and the discord actually represents an effort to reestablish this emotional connection. Until emotional connectivity is reestablished and the reactive fear of losing it is quelled, standard couples counseling techniques will be futile. Healthy couples do not problem-solve or communicate in any particularly unique way. Although necessary, simply discontinuing unhealthy patterns does not generate emotional connectivity. Not only are standard counseling techniques ineffective at reestablishing connection, they often increase the distance between partners and reconfirm fears of loss, rejection, and abandonment.

Couples who engage in counseling should look for a practitioner who possesses an approach of healing emotional wounding and attachment panic rather than the usual approach of changing behaviors. A third party should not inject themselves into your relationship to determine who was right and who was wrong in your disagreements. Therapists who take sides and make determinations about arguments will leave one party feeling defeated while the other feels victorious. Relationships should be win-win, not win-lose.

Types of Abuse

Partners can perpetrate various types of abuse, knowingly or unknowingly. Abuse covers a variety of behaviors including physical abuse, verbal abuse, sexual abuse, financial abuse, emotional abuse, and emotional neglect. All forms of abuse have an underlying dynamic of gaining and maintaining power and control. Abuse is never acceptable and there is no excuse for abusing a partner or tolerating abuse.

When people hear the term "abuse," most people think of physical abuse, which encompasses a wide range of behaviors, from shoving, spitting, and slapping to physical beatings. Physical abuse behaviors tend to begin gradually and partners may rationalize physical abuse, especially if it does not result in injury. Examples include: pulling your hair, grabbing your clothing, slapping your behind without consent or in a non-playful way, grabbing your face, covering your mouth, pushing, and shoving. Other threatening or intimidating behaviors such as gestures with a weapon or restricting your movement can also be considered physical abuse.

Verbal abuse extends beyond yelling and name-calling. It may also include judging, criticizing, accusing, blaming, dismissing, minimizing, undermining, and demanding. Teasing and joking can rise to the level of verbal abuse, especially in front of others when the outcome creates the appearance of inferiority. Threatening is another common form of verbal abuse.

Sexual abuse includes behaviors beyond sexual assault. Coercing a partner to be sexually intimate or to participate in activities to which they object by threatening to leave the relationship is abusive. Criticizing a partner's sexual performance or preferences is also abusive.

Financial abuse is a type of relationship abuse that is often overlooked. Behaviors that would be considered financial abuse include imposing an allowance, monitoring a partner's spending without their own accountability, hiding money or financial records, forbidding a partner from working or keeping their own money, destroying a partner's credit or perpetrating identity theft, stealing a partner's money or credit cards, using children's education or savings accounts, being financially irresponsible or failing to pay household bills.

Emotional abuse constitutes behaviors that harm another person emotionally. Common forms of emotional abuse include manipulation and guilt-inducing statements, as well as gaslighting, which is a behavior that causes a person to question themselves in some way. Withholding, failing to share thoughts or feelings, or shutting down, can also be considered emotional abuse.

Emotional neglect includes failing to be emotionally supportive and meeting a partner's emotional needs. Emotional neglect can be insidious in relationships because it is difficult for many people to articulate that which is missing. Neglect is the absence of something. It often presents as "we don't communicate with each other" and "I feel lonely in my relationship."

Cheating

Of all the choices we make in life, cheating is one we should reconsider more than any other. Cheating is deeply devastating to the person who was betrayed, rarely accomplishes the intended goal (whether it is to fulfill a physical need or to fix a deep-rooted problem in the relationship), and creates more problems than it solves. Cheating undermines the fundamental relationship pillar of trust.

First, let's explore what constitutes cheating. Cheating is not just sexual contact. It can include such behaviors as emotional relationships with friends or coworkers, watching porn, going to strip clubs, as well as online flirting and relationships. Behaviors that violate the relationship boundary are a betrayal. Think of a bubble existing around the relationship. A simple rule of thumb to follow is to ask yourself if you would do what you are doing if your partner were standing next to you. If the answer is no, consider the behavior a betrayal that has the potential to burst the relationship bubble. Another simple rule of thumb is to ask yourself how you would feel if the situation was reversed. Would it be hurtful? If the answer is yes, the behavior is a betrayal.

So, if cheating is so devastating, why do people cheat? There are various reasons for cheating. Immaturity often leads to cheating. Many people desire the benefits of being in a relationship but do not understand the consequences of cheating or they fail to view the relationship through a lens of commitment. People with immature relationship skills often have few tools at their disposal and also seek immediate need – satisfaction/gratification. Other issues such as addiction and impulsivity can contribute to cheating. Insecurity and the need for external validation and reassurance, as well as selfishness can contribute to betrayals. Cheating is a solution with a singular focus on the self.

Terminal uniqueness involves the belief that an individual is different and special in some way and therefore deserves the benefits of cheating that do not apply to other people. Individuals may also convince themselves about the intensity of their feelings for someone else when the relationship is new, thereby confusing romantic love, or limerence, with commitment. These new feelings, although intoxicating, do not replace the deeper, more meaningful connections of long-term relationships.

Before the commencement of any cheating behaviors, consider the dynamics outlined. Recovering from infidelity is a long and difficult process. Because the person who perpetrated the betrayal does not also feel the deep, intense pain of the other partner, the process of recovery is arduous. For those struggling with the after-effects of cheating, review Day 20, Repairing Wounds.

First Steps to Healing

For purposes of today's lesson, relationship difficulties do not include domestic violence or drug use. In relationships where domestic violence or drug use is present, outside help must be sought. These issues cannot be healed inside of the relationship by two partners.

In the midst of relationship discord, many people feel unheard and resort to escalating tactics to feel heard, such as yelling and manipulation. It is common for most people wait for their partner to change and believe that the relationship can only improve once their partner is "fixed."

The first step in healing the wounds in a relationship is to make the decision to do something different. The definition of insanity is doing the same thing and expecting a different result. Improving your relationship is no different. You must be different in the relationship in order to have a different relationship.

After you have made the decision to change your mindset, attitude, and approach toward your partner, the best place to begin is by learning to hear your partner, followed by validating and empathizing with your partner. Remember, your partner is waiting for you to change as much as you are waiting for your partner to change. Begin giving your partner what you want to receive. To begin to hear your partner, use healthy communication skills (learned on Day 9) and address behaviors and feelings. If your partner addresses any particular issue with you, instead of explaining or rationalizing, try simply hearing your partner. Hearing your partner includes summarizing, rephrasing, and repeating back what you have heard. For example, your partner tells you that he hates it when you are on your phone instead of listening to him. A typical response for most people is, "You do the same thing to me." Instead, try, "So, you're unhappy when I'm on my phone because I'm not listening to you very well."

Next, try validating and empathizing with your partner. Validation is powerful because it lets your partner know that you accept what they feel. The beauty of validation is that you do not need to be in agreement. Partners do not have identical emotional experiences. An example of validating is, "It makes sense that you are unhappy with that behavior. I get it." Adding empathy to the conversation is healing and connecting. Empathy is the process of understanding or feeling the emotional experience of another person. An example of empathy includes, "It makes me sad and I feel a little guilty that something that I am doing makes you unhappy." Notice the lack of apology. Apologies do not provide assurances that the behavior will change.

Empathy is key because it creates connectedness. It is the process of truly listening and being available to your partner. It is a calming experience and it changes the dynamic from combatant to partner.

Another helpful exercise is to create a list of rules of engagement for the relationship. If your partner is not on board with creating a list, you can create a list by yourself for yourself. Some examples include:

Use healthy communication
No name-calling
No blaming
No criticizing
No yelling
Remain on topic
Do not bring up past events
Use time-outs instead of walking away

Avoid shutting down
Use validation and empathy
Agree to revisit the argument if it cannot be resolved
Do not threaten divorce
Do not use hurtful information against my partner
No use of alcohol or drugs
Do not go to bed angry
Respect physical boundaries

Use the following chart to create your own list:

RULES OF ENGAGEMENT FOR OUR RELATIONSHIP:

HOMEWORK DAY 27

QUOTE OF THE DAY:

*THE HEART THAT BREAKS OPEN CAN CONTAIN THE WHOLE
UNIVERSE. – JOANNA MACY*

1) Complete Elements for a Healthy Relationship assessment.
   Practice First Steps to Healing (Hearing, Validation, and Empathy) exercise.
   Complete Rules of Engagement list.

2) Identify daily gratitude.

3) Conduct exposure therapy and take a break from ABC worksheets.

4) Make a commitment to complete Day 28.

YOU CAN DO IT! YOU'VE DONE INCREDIBLE WORK SO FAR!!!

DAY 28 PARENTING SKILLS

Today's Objectives: 1) Learn basic parenting principles 2) Learn what attunement is and why it is important for parenting 3) Learn the concept of consequence parenting 4) Begin to implement consequence parenting

A discussion about parenting may seem out of place, however, parenting skills that lead to frustration (on the part of the adult and the child) can have a profound effect on mental health and well-being. Ineffective parenting skills have negative effects on children's mental well-being, peer relationships, future adult relationships, and their own parenting style.

The main objective for today's lesson is to learn to parent on purpose. When we parent on purpose, we parent *with* purpose. Much like the other lessons, today's lesson aims to help you alter reactive patterns of functioning. Many parenting interactions occur on a reactive basis, in that way, they emanate from the parent's emotional state. Reactive parenting results in frustration, yelling, and punishing parent-child interactions. Reactive responses reflect poor parenting skills that lead to low self-esteem in children and depressive and anxiety symptoms in adulthood.

In today's lesson, you will learn some basic parenting concepts and some basic skills to help you build an effective parenting toolbox and skill set. For those who are not parents, these skills will benefit you with nieces, nephews, other children with whom you relate, or your future children.

Attunement

The first concept important to effective parenting is attunement, which is the awareness of the needs, thoughts, and emotions of another person, as well as the ability to respond appropriately. Most needs, thoughts, and emotions are not communicated directly, but rather, indirectly, through facial expressions, non-verbal signals, posture, and environmental cues.

Attunement between a parent and a child is important for the purpose of meeting the needs of the child. Significantly, attunement is also the foundation on which the child builds its sense of self and its concept of the world. A child with an attuned caregiver will feel loved, important, valued, and worthy. The child will learn that the world is safe and will enthusiastically learn and explore. It is the job of a child's primary caregiver to be attuned and fulfill this crucial role in a child's development. A child with a caregiver who is not attuned will emotionally and behaviorally suffer. A child who cannot predict the attunement of their primary caregiver will experience anxiety about having its core needs met.

Attunement is crucial for social development in a child. A child who experiences healthy attunement will have the ability to develop strong attachments to others and will have an innate ability to form healthy social relationships with others as they explore the world. Children develop from their primary caregivers an understanding of how to respond in various social situations. The confidence a child needs for healthy development and functioning is formed through attunement and attachment.

Children with attuned caregivers develop confidence, self-awareness, and good self-esteem. These children tend to have few emotional vulnerabilities and are able to tolerate stressful emotions and social situations. They are adaptable and respond well to changes in their environment.

Attunement is best started in infancy but it is never too late to attune to a child. Nature automatically gives us the skill of attunement. Think about a baby smiling and cooing at its mother. The mother's automatic and instinctual response is to mimic the baby with the same smile and the same cooing sound.

These interactions between parent and baby send a message of attunement. It signals to the baby that they can trust that the caregiver is present and will tend to the baby's needs, which is crucial for survival. Because this process begins at birth and becomes hard-wired in the brain, attunement with those around us arouses a primal message of safety.

For infants, attunement strategies enable parents to provide more responsive parenting. Begin by being as present as possible when interacting with your baby. Giving undivided attention, establishing eye contact, following facial expressions, imitating vocalizations, and mirroring body movements can all send messages of attunement and safety. Consciously practicing these activities on a daily basis will establish a soothing, nurturing relationship for the infant.

For toddlers, activities that can be done together, such as coloring, finger painting, and crafting can be excellent opportunities to enhance the parent-child bond. Activities that involve taking turns, such as using blocks or Legos present an opportunity for mirroring. Dancing presents a unique opportunity for mirroring and attunement as the adult mimics the child's moves.

Attunement is an important concept to continue as the child grows and also serves us well in other relationships, such as family, friends, and intimate partners. Attunement in adult relationships sends messages of connection, value, and safety. These strategies enhance and strengthen relationships by signaling a sense of respect, resulting in greater satisfaction for both partners.

Parenting on Purpose

Every interaction a parent has with a child influences who they become as a person. Think of each experience with a child as a learning opportunity and a chance to shape who they are. Each experience will not be perfect, or even positive, but we can set a goal to minimize the negative impact on the child's development.

Begin by considering how you speak to your child. Words are powerful tools. Labels become part of our belief system and individuals have a tendency to act in accordance with what is expected of them. We tend to incorporate labels into our identity. A child who is told that they are the "smart one" will tend to see themselves as smart and fulfill that role. Labels have the ability to shape personality and shape our relationships with others.

Below is a list of guidelines to help you begin parenting on purpose:

1. Remember to interact with your child on an age-appropriate level. Toddlers are not little adults and it is the job of the parent to know what a child is capable of understanding.

2. Set your expectations at an age-appropriate level. Children do not have the life experiences of an adult and have a limited frame of reference for many situations.

3. Minimize use of the word 'no' as much as possible. Tell your child what it is that you want them to do instead of what you don't want them to do. Instead of telling a child to stop jumping on the sofa, tell the child to sit down and put their feet forward.

4. Model manners for your child. If you want your child to use manners and treat others with respect, model it with your child. When your child hands you something, say thank you to engrain in them the use of please and thank you.

5. Model behaviors for your child. If you want your child to treat their belongings with respect, don't slam the kitchen drawers and expect your child to be gentle with their toys.

6. Try to find a teachable moment in daily events. If a child accidently breaks a glass, teach the child about being careful and teach them how to clean up broken glass.

7. Use open-ended questions about anything in their world to encourage communication. Children who are used to talking to their parents about what they built with Legos in great detail turn into teenagers who tell their parents details about their lives. As we listen to our children, they learn that they are important and that what they say matters.

8. Assist children with understanding anger and model problem-solving skills. Adults usually try to eliminate a child's anger. An angry person who is told to stop being angry only becomes angrier! Think about being frustrated at work and a coworker comes along and tells you that they would be mad at the situation as well. Validation is important for children. It helps them learn to understand their emotions, which is the beginning of learning to manage them.

9. Allow children to manage their own problems and emotional responses. Children need to learn to tolerate frustration and learn how to problem-solve. Children deprived of learning these skills are developmentally disadvantaged.

10. Allow children to experience consequences. Consequences correlate with age. The younger we are, the smaller the consequences. The older we get, the bigger the consequences. As a child, the consequence of hitting a sibling is a time out. The consequence of hitting as an adult is an assault charge.

Consequence Parenting

Consequence parenting is a way of parenting that teaches a child to self-monitor, self-regulate, and develop a conscience. It teaches children to learn right from wrong. Parenting becomes a positive experience and it significantly reduces anxiety and frustration on the part of the parent and the child.

Consequences are a natural part of life. When a child chooses a behavior, they choose the consequence. As adults, we are free to choose our behaviors, but we are not free from the consequences. When you use consequence parenting, children learn that they have power and control over their worlds and they learn to choose good behaviors for intrinsic reasons. Consequence parenting teaches children right from wrong and teaches them to have a conscience, as well as to think for themselves.

To begin, choose a child's top five behavioral issues. With input from the child, choose a natural, short-term consequence for each behavior. Children are more likely to participate and buy into the process when they play a role in the choices for behaviors and consequences. For example, the behavior of not completing homework may have a consequence of not watching television for the evening. When you identify behaviors, remember the following:

1. Choose behaviors, not traits. Do not choose 'being lazy.'

2. Encourage the child's participation. If they do not want to participate, let them know that the consequences will be imposed with or without their input.

3. Have the child write down the behaviors and the consequences. A chart on a poster board is a great visual reminder for kids. Post the chart where everyone can see it. When you refer to the chart, have the child go to the chart and identify what behavior is being addressed.

4. Allow the child to pick their poster board. Most kids like bright colors. Allow them to decorate it with drawings and stickers.

5. Choose consequences that are immediate.

6. Choose consequences that are short-term in nature and are not open-ended. For example, do not take your child's video game for an extended period of time, until you feel like giving it back, or when they "decide to act right."

7. Choose consequences you can live with. If you cannot follow through with taking your child's phone, choose another consequence.

8. Do not choose consequences that require the child to do something. It is easier to select a consequence that you can control, such as no television, versus having the child empty the dishwasher.

9. Create a chart for yourself. Children love to have a chart for the adults and it helps them to buy into the process even further. When an adult follows through with a consequence for a behavior, it makes it more difficult for the child to argue when it is time to experience their own consequence.

Begin to implement consequence parenting by creating your own chart with your child(ren). Review the example for ideas. The chart is not carved in stone and is meant to be changed as problematic behaviors are remediated and as the child ages.

BEHAVIOR	CONSEQUENCE
Homework not done by 7 p.m.	No television for 24 hours
Not ready to leave house by 7:05 a.m. on school days	Bedtime is 30 minutes earlier that night
Hitting sibling	No electronics for 24 hours and apologize
Cursing	No electronics for 24 hours Child must restate what he/she said without curse word
Forget to take trash out Monday evenings	No cell phone for 24 hours

BEHAVIOR	CONSEQUENCE

HOMEWORK DAY 28

1) Complete Consequence Parenting chart.

2) Identify daily gratitude.

3) Conduct exposure therapy and take a break from ABC worksheets.

4) Make a commitment to complete Day 29.

ALMOST THERE!!!

DAY 29 MINDFULNESS

Today's Objectives: 1) Learn about mindfulness 2) Discover the benefits of mindfulness 3) Learn ways to implement mindfulness techniques to improve mental health

In today's lesson, we will explore the concept of mindfulness, which is a type of meditation. Mindfulness has existed for thousands of years and finds its origins in Eastern cultures. Mindfulness, like many Eastern practices, is experiencing a resurgence in recent years as people discover their intrinsic benefits.

What is mindfulness? Mindfulness consists of three main concepts: awareness, present experience, acceptance. It involves bringing your consciousness to the present moment and experience it without judgment. Mindfulness does not judge the experience, but rather, observes the experience.

There are a number of misconceptions about mindfulness. For instance, mindfulness practice does not involve relaxation, although it can be relaxing. Relaxation is not the end goal of mindfulness exercises. Mindfulness is not used for avoidance, nor is it a way to alter your state of mind. Mindfulness is not used for clearing your mind to reach a state of thoughtlessness. Rather, mindfulness exercises are about being an observer of your thoughts, emotions, and sensations without judgment. In a world wrought with judgement, considering your thoughts and feelings without judgment can be a cleansing and clarifying experience. It can also be very liberating.

Mindfulness is not problem-solving oriented. The goal is not about finding solutions – it is about finding acceptance. Remember, what you resist, persists. What you accept, transforms.

Mindfulness may sound corny but there are many benefits to regular practice. Mindfulness eases anxiety because the brain learns it is not necessary to avoid what the brain naturally wants to avoid, such as painful memories and unpleasant emotions. Regular exercises will result in an increased ability to tolerate unpleasant emotions, thoughts, and sensations. Mindfulness can have a positive impact on anxiety. Remember, when we avoid unpleasant memories, thoughts, and feelings, they intensify over time.

Mindfulness can also ease depression because it teaches acceptance. Depression can improve because it removes gap between how things are in any given moment and how we wish them to be. That gap is often a source of depression. As we learn to accept without judgment, negative thinking patterns such as jumping to conclusions and catastrophizing will remediate.

Mindfulness allows us to stop living life on autopilot. The daily gratitude exercises over the last few weeks are a good start for increased mindfulness. Practicing these exercises will allow you to learn to live in present moment without distress and to live in an enjoyable way.

Mindfulness can also have a positive impact on sleep, especially falling asleep, as the brain learns to refrain from ruminating thoughts. As the brain learns to be calm, it is easier to fall asleep.

Mindfulness has seven key components:

COMPONENT	
Breathing	Focus on the sound and the rate of your natural breath
Thoughts	Allow thoughts to come and go without judgment
Mantra	Develop a mantra such as "I will accept these feelings even if they are unpleasant" or "I can have a thought without reacting"
Body sensations	Notice any tightness or tingling and let it pass
Sensory	Become aware of sounds, sights, smells, or tastes
Emotions	Put a word to any emotion you feel and be aware of it without judgment
Urge surfing	Notice any craving and focus on not being reactive

As you begin to practice, take note of whether the aspect of mindfulness you experience is internal or external. Internal components include breathing, thoughts, bodily sensations, and emotions. Examples of external parts include sensory elements such as what you see or what you hear. During your exercise, incorporate elements in each category.

Mindfulness can be practiced informally or formally. Examples of informal practice include the awareness of any physical habit such as holding the steering wheel, awareness of your breathing, awareness of your voice during communications. Consider becoming more aware of your morning routine or the details and sensations of completing domestic chores.

More formal mindfulness includes taking time out during your day to practice. With the increasing demands on our time, it is difficult for many people to devote time to such endeavors. For those who choose to formally practice, scheduling a specific time every day, as well as creating a plan of how the practice will be conducted will ensure success.

There are several methods to begin to implement mindfulness into your life. Several methods to keep in mind as you begin your mindfulness journey include:

Go with the flow. Go with the flow is the practice of observing without judgment. Observing can be difficult and takes some practice in order to master it, as emotional responses can be intense and it is your brain's inclination to make sense of what you are experiencing, which is expressed as judging the experience.

Pay attention. Paying attention to our internal and external sensations follows the ability to observe without judgment.

Stay with it. Once we are able to observe and become aware of thoughts, emotions, and sensations, you will develop an increasing ability to stay with mindfulness with practice. It is difficult at first but becomes easier over time as you become increasingly comfortable with the components.

It is likely that your mind will wander or get stuck in negative thoughts and worries. Gently redirecting your attention without judgment will bring your awareness back to the present.

Just like any other skill, repetition is key to better practice. Consider any other skill you learn. The first time you ride a bike or play tennis, you will not be proficient. After a while, your skill level will improve. Mindfulness is no different. If you miss a session or have a bad session, just continue to practice.

The final step to learning mindfulness is to implement it. Following are some ways to practice mindfulness. Try them and use the one that works most effectively for you. You may use more than one method or change your method with time.

1) Take 10 deep breaths. Notice your thoughts and your feelings. Concentrate on observing without judgment.

2) Notice 5 things you can see, 5 things you can hear, 5 things you can feel in contact with your body. For example, be aware of the watch on your wrist, the shoes on your feet, the air on your face, and the sensation of the chair you are sitting in.

3) For one minute each, notice 1) what you feel in your body (with your eyes closed), 2) what you see, 3) what images you have in your mind (with your eyes closed), and 4) what you hear (with your eyes closed).

4) Become aware of the practice of avoiding 'just worrying.' Begin by differentiating between worrying and problem-solving. Worrying is circular, provides no solution, and relates to anxiety symptoms. Identify worrying thoughts; bring your attention to your breath, current sensations, and your current environment; and move into acceptance. The idea is not about changing from 'just worrying' to 'don't worry' – the idea is not to change but to increase non-judgmental awareness and acceptance. This practice also works with 'just doubting' and 'just criticizing.'

HOMEWORK DAY 29

QUOTE OF THE DAY:

WITHOUT RAIN NOTHING GROWS. LEARN TO ACCEPT THE STORMS
IN YOUR LIFE. - UNKNOWN

1) Choose a mindfulness exercise and practice it.

2) Identify daily gratitude.

3) Conduct exposure therapy and complete a *final* (for this Boot Camp) ABC worksheet on any situation.

4) Make a commitment to complete the last day!

ONE MORE DAY! YOU CAN DO IT!!!

DAY 30 FORGIVENESS

Today's Objective: 1) Learn about forgiveness concepts 2) Learn the myths about forgiveness that lead to distress 3) Learn how to implement forgiveness

In today's final lesson, we will discuss forgiveness. It is not an accident that forgiveness is at the end of the book and not at the beginning. It is common lore that forgiveness is the key to healing and moving forward from hurt and tragedy.

For those who have been victimized or betrayed in the form of a friend's lie or deceit, a cheating partner, a crime victim, or a horrific tragedy, the prospect of forgiving can feel overwhelming and seemingly impossible. It is natural, healthy, and necessary to feel and fully experience your emotions and to process aspects of the event before forgiveness is possible. Forgiveness is a process and not a destination.

The cognitive process of ABC Worksheets from Day 1 and the exercise from Day 25, Narrative Therapy, is a good start for healing wounds, big or small. Understanding forgiveness is also crucial for being able to begin the process of forgiving.

First, let's look at what forgiveness is. Forgiveness is the process of letting something go. That something may be the need for justice or the need for revenge. Even in cases where revenge comes to fruition, it does not make right what was wrong. In fact, it often serves to perpetuate or intensify the pain of the original event. Revenge may feel triumphant in the moment but is most likely to be followed with sadness and defeat. Revenge causes a person to act in a way that is not congruent with their own integrity, which can be disconcerting rather than healing.

Forgiveness is also the ability to release negative thoughts of bitterness and resentment. Again, ABC Worksheets from Day 1, as well as the exercise from Day 23, Reframe Loss to Gain, assist with the process of addressing negative thoughts and creating new, healthier thought processes.

Finally, forgiveness is the process of giving up something to which we have a moral right. Sometimes the moral right is the right to be hurt or angry and sometimes it is the right to be compensated for damages or harm. Remember that forgiveness is a gift for the person doing the forgiving, it is not for the perpetrator.

The most common misperception about forgiveness is that it is a gift that is given to the other person. Oftentimes, the other person is unaware of the hurt, does not care about being forgiven, or may no longer exist.

Now, let's take a look at what forgiveness is not. Forgiveness does not diminish the wrong nor does it condone it. Forgiveness is not about enabling wrongdoing, denying wrongdoing, or waiting for an apology (which will likely never come). Forgiveness does not involve forgetting, neglecting justice, restoring trust, or reconciliation with the perpetrator. Forgiveness is also not a singular event, and it will not eliminate the pain of the original offense. Forgiveness is not easy and requires work on ourselves, for ourselves.

Remember, forgiveness is not for another person. It is a gift that we give to ourselves to set us free from being tied to pain. When we are finally able to contemplate forgiveness, we can begin the process of letting something go. Often what is let go is the need for revenge, which never rights the wrong.

Forgiveness allows for the release of negative thoughts of bitterness and resentment. As demonstrated in several of the lessons in this book, learning how to identify, address, and change negative thoughts is an important skill to learn in order to progress to a state of healing where forgiveness is possible. Our power lies in our ability to develop command of our thoughts and our emotions. Having that power is the key to healing because past events cannot change.

Finally, the path to forgiveness also includes the process of giving up something to which we have a moral right, which is the right to be hurt or angry. Holding on to hurt and anger harms no one but ourselves. Carrying the burden of hurt and anger is a heavy weight that we choose to carry and we have the option to put it down. Forgiveness is a voluntary thought process, not a feeling. Many people spend their lives waiting for the feeling of forgiveness to wash over them. Since forgiveness is a process, not a destination, that event is unlikely.

Use the following forgiveness worksheet to assist with the process.

FORGIVENESS AND ACCEPTANCE WORKSHEET

1. Identify the hurt, injury, or damage that occurred. It can be anything, no matter how small or large.

2. List the ways you benefit from having these unresolved negative feelings.

3. List the ways you are negatively affected by these feelings.

4. Admit that you cannot change what has happened, and own that the lingering feelings are yours to resolve. Identify what you say to yourself to accept that these feelings that negatively affect you are yours to fix (for your own sake).

5. Choose forgiveness. If possible, use perspective and empathize with the other party.

HOMEWORK DAY 30

FALL SEVEN TIMES, STAND UP EIGHT. – JAPANESE PROVERB

1) Complete Forgiveness Worksheet.

2) Identify daily gratitude.

3) Conduct exposure therapy and continue until anxiety subsides substantially.

4) Make a commitment to continue to use the skills learned in this book and have a great life!

DONE! YOU SHOULD BE EXTREMELY PROUD OF YOURSELF! TIME FOR A LIFE OF PEACE AND CONTENTMENT!!!